THE ART OF HEALING

THE ART OF HEALING

CHRONIC ILLNESSES

OBESITY AND

ADDICTIONS

WITH

DIET

NUTRITION AND

ALTERNATIVE MEDICINE.

DR. GARY J. SHIMA, MD

MARC S. HERLANDS, JD

Library of Congress Control Number:		2014902816
ISBN:	Hardcover	978-1-4931-7322-8
	Softcover	978-1-4931-7323-5
	eBook	978-1-4931-7324-2

Printed in the United States of America by BookMasters, Inc
Ashland OH
September 2014

Rev. date: 05/30/2014

To order additional copies of this book, contact:
Xlibris LLC
1-888-795-4274
www.Xlibris.com
Orders@Xlibris.com
553402

CONTENTS

Chronic Illnesses

Obesity

Alcoholism

Chronic Fatigue Syndrome

Fibromyalgia

Celiac Disease

Depression

Rheumatoid Arthritis

Gulf War Syndrome

Mycoplasma

Heavy-Metal Toxicity / Poisoning

Chronic Yeast Infection

Chronic Viral Infections

With Spiritual Insights for the Chronically Ill

Using traditional, complementary, and alternative therapies, including

vitamin, mineral, and amino-acid enhancements;

enzyme enhancements;

celiac disease regulation with diet and nutrients;

yeast and fungus control for CFS, fibromyalgia, obesity and alcoholism;

colon hydrotherapy / colonics for CFS and fibromyalgia;

chelation for CFS and fibromyalgia;

colloidal silver and antibiotics for mycoplasma and
    Gulf War Syndrome;

antibiotics for rheumatoid arthritis;

special medicines for CFS and fibromyalgia;

prolotherapy for fibromyalgia;

marijuana for fibromyalgia;

special exercises for lymph cleaning, CFS and fibromyalgia;

immune system regulation for CFS and fibromyalgia;

meditation;

mental focusing techniques;

prayer and surrender.

To My Wife and My Other Angels

To my dearest wife, Louise L. Herlands—affectionately known to me as Louie or Lou—the love of my life for thirty years, who never gave up on me and always encouraged me on my journey to recovery. God bless you and your memory.

And to all my other angels, including my friends, family, doctors, dentists, health-care practitioners, and supporters, who gave me their unyielding love and understanding on my long journey back to health.

I wish to acknowledge all of you and thank you with my life and my love.

Disclaimer

Dear Reader: The information provided in this book is *for informational purposes only*. It is *not* to be construed as *medical advice* or *medical care*, and the information herein is *not* a replacement for professional medical advice or care given by licensed physicians or trained medical personnel. The author and publisher do *not* directly or indirectly *practice* medicine. Nor do they dispense medical advice, care, diagnosis, treatment, or any other medical service.

Dear Patient: *Always* seek the advice of your physician or other qualified health-care provider whenever you experience symptoms or health problems, or before starting any new medical treatment. Please note that the author and publisher are *not* responsible for any inaccuracies, omissions, or editorial errors in this book; or for any consequences resulting from the information provided herein.

Dear Physician: It is always *your* responsibility to evaluate the information provided herein and the results from the information provided.

Dear Health-Care Professional: You should always exercise your professional judgment when evaluating any information provided herein. We *encourage* you to confirm from other sources that the information provided herein is accurate in all respects *before* undertaking any treatment protocol or any other action that may be based upon the information presented herein.

Statement by Gary J. Shima, MD

I have been Marc Herland's primary care physician for twenty-two years. He was the type of patient I have come to enjoy working with over my many years of medical practice. After forty-three years of practicing medicine, I am not accepting any new patients.

I began practicing medicine in California in 1968. Since then and to the present, I have treated numerous patients for all sorts of disorders, including the chronically ill patient.

During my many years of practice, I came to realize that *health* and *longevity* were two of my most persistent interests as a treating physician.

To help my patients accomplish these goals, I frequently prescribed that my patients make significant changes in their dietary and exercise habits, fortify themselves with additional vitamins, minerals, and amino acids, and use other approved remedial health techniques.

Over time, I came to believe that using therapies as described in this book in conjunction with standard medicines were appropriate to help many of my chronically ill patients recover from their illnesses.

As a medical doctor, I have used standardized medical testing, practice, and protocols. But I have also used other techniques that have met the California Medical Board's standards of ethical medical practice.

I have ordered various methods of testing, both standard and nonstandard, and I have used and ordered various methods of treatments, both standard and nonstandard, many of which are listed in this book.

Depending upon the health and vitality of the patient, the results ranged from spectacular to not productive. But in fairness, almost everyone received some benefit, and most patients received significant benefits from their treatments.

Marc Herlands is an example of one of my many challenging patients. He presented himself with many medical problems that had obscure causes and where the remedies were not readily apparent. He has given me permission to fully discuss his case.

He first came to me for help in 1991. I had recently opened an office in Encinitas, California, with William Kellas, PhD, which is now called the Center for Advanced Medicine and is presently under the medical supervision of Mark Drucker, MD.

In that office, I treated patients who had complicated illnesses, or were chronically ill, and for most, there were no obvious causes for their illnesses.

At that time, Marc presented himself to me with symptoms of great depression, suicidal ideation, chronic fatigue to the point of chronic exhaustion, chronic muscle pain, morbid obesity, swollen lymph glands in his neck, and major sleep disorder.

He came to me with a history of hypothyroidism, hypoglycemia, a melanoma on his back, long-term depression, and an episode of admission to a hospital emergency room due to an obstructed bowel caused by severe constipation.

He told me that for the previous two years, he had been unable to work in any capacity as an attorney because he suffered from severe memory and cognitive disorders. He said that he did not know of any causes for his illnesses.

As his primary physician, I started by taking his medical and family history and gave him a brief physical exam, none of which indicated any obvious causes for his illnesses.

I then ordered a series of standard medical tests to determine the general state of his health. The results appeared normal except for some abnormalities in his immune system, and he had a low level of infection.

I ordered further testing of his immune system and testing to determine the cause of his infection. As I remember, the results indicated that he was suffering from immune system dysfunction, and he tested positive for cytomegalic viral infection. These factors could have explained the causes of many of his symptoms.

The plan I established was to regulate his immune system and cure the infection. I ordered him to use vitamin and mineral supplements to increase his vitality and to use transfer factor injections three times per week. The injections were prepared by an immunologist and administered by the nursing staff at my office.

After three months, Marc reported that his energy improved a little, his fatigue was reduced a little, but he was still not feeling well. None of his other problems had been reduced.

After a further review of his preliminary testing, I concluded that he might be suffering from heavy-metal toxicity. Thus, I ordered a medical chelation test to determine the level of heavy metals in his body.

The results were astounding because his tests revealed that he had accumulated very high levels of lead, mercury, nickel, vanadium, and cadmium.

After discussing the results with him, we determined that nothing in Marc's environment or recent activities could account for these levels of heavy metals. I concluded that, most probably, he had accumulated these metals by being exposed to them during the course of his lifetime, and his body had not excreted a sufficient amount, which resulted in the accumulation of large amounts of heavy metals.

To reduce the levels of heavy metals, I ordered for Marc, as treatment therapy, chelation IV infusions twice per week in addition to one electrolyte replacement IV infusion per week.

At first, the treatments seemed to help him quite a bit. But after nine weeks, his illnesses began to worsen. By the eighteenth week, the chelation treatments had become too exhausting for him to continue.

Convinced that a significant portion of his problems stemmed from his body's accumulation of heavy metals, and with no obvious way to rid them from his body, I ordered that he use colon hydrotherapy.

He reported that he immediately felt better from the first treatment. So I ordered that he continue with that course of treatment. He stayed on the course for the next nine years.

During the next twenty-two years, Marc presented himself to me with many other interesting and unusual illnesses. One was particularly noteworthy: he had contracted an infection from *Mycoplasma fermentans incognitus*. I ordered a culture from a lab, which determined that he had such an infection.

Over the course of the next few months, I developed a protocol to rid his body of that infectious agent. A subsequent lab culture confirmed that he had gotten rid of that infectious agent.

Unfortunately, many years later, he contracted the disease of mycoplasma again. The next time, I ordered that he use colloidal silver injections to help kill that infectious agent.

Another important underlying aspect of Marc's illnesses was his infection from yeast and fungus. He responded well to an anti-yeast and fungus diet as well as to the use of antifungal medication.

In conclusion, this book is obviously intended for general informational purposes only, and it is not to be used in any manner for diagnostic or treatment purposes.

It should only be used in conjunction with a qualified medical practitioner who is licensed by the state or country in which the patient seeks medical advice or treatment.

The opinions in the book are Marc's, but I have read the book, and I do not have any objections to what it contains.

During my years of medical practice, I have used most of the treatment protocols presented in this book. Therefore, I can generally endorse the effectiveness of the treatments presented in this book when used under proper medical supervision and with the appropriate patient.

I consider that the medical tests listed in this book are an excellent source of information when researching possible causes of chronic illnesses.

I found that, many times, one or more of the tests listed in this book provided an important clue for discovering what were the underlying causes of my patient's chronic illnesses.

I found that once the causes of the patient's illnesses were discovered, the appropriate course of medical treatment became apparent.

I believe this book contains valuable information for the chronically ill patient.

I feel fortunate that I have been able to help Marc and so many other chronically ill patients recover from their illnesses during my long medical career.

Gary J. Shima, MD
Medical Director
Health and Longevity Institute
San Marcos, California

Preface

You may have noticed that this book has large print, wide margins, and extra space between paragraphs. It was created like this on purpose because it was written to include a specific group of people. It was written for those who need to take extensive notes about what they have just read.

As a proud member of this group, let me share that we need wide margins and extra space to write our thoughts and questions *immediately* as they come to us. Otherwise, we soon forget what we were thinking about.

This book uses large print, simple language, and basic sentence structure because we have significant difficulties reading, comprehending, and remembering what we read.

People with cognitive challenges or "brain fog" know why I did this and appreciate my efforts.

Those who have *empathy* for our problems—our doctors, medical advisors, healers, caregivers, coworkers, bosses, friends, and family—understand these things and appreciate my efforts to accommodate as well.

But those who do not know us very well do not grasp the great medical challenges we face every day because we have brain fog.

So I have to explain these things to those people who don't have or never have had any problems with thinking, reading, comprehending, or remembering.

If you find yourself thinking this book is too simple and you should discount the information contained herein, please consider that as a member of Mensa, my IQ was measured to be in the top 2 percent of the population, and I have earned a general law degree and a master's degree in tax law.

It is not that I am unintelligent. It is that I am writing to include people who have big challenges with cognition.

If you do not have or never have had any of these problems, consider yourself very lucky.

People who have these challenges have it rough—physically, mentally, emotionally, and financially.

It is for them I have written this book.

It is for them my heart bleeds.

Acknowledgments

My very special thanks to

Gary Shima, MD
Health and Longevity Institute
1529 Grand Avenue, Suite B
San Marcos, CA 92078

and

Ms. Roxanne Watson, CHT
Living Water Rejuvenation Center
5670 El Camino Real
Carlsbad, CA 92008
www.LivingWaterRejuvenation.com

and

Ms. Cathy Brady, JD, LLM
Mark Drucker, MD
Ms. Svetlana Elbert, BS

Hal Huggins, DDS
Ronald Lesko, DO
William Kellas, PhD
Javier Morales, DDS
Garth Nicolson, PhD
Mr. Mark J. Olsen, AF
R. Paul St. Amand, MD
Mr. Dennis Schiller, BA
Ms. Shirley Smith, AS
Mr. William Timmons, ND

All of whom played a direct and very important part in saving my life since 1991.

We would be remiss without thanking Paul Lloyd Warner for his wonderful contributions to the book's layout and design, and Anthony R. Neenan for his great assistance with editorial content and project management.

Introduction

The Art of Healing Chronic Illnesses, Obesity, and Addictions with Diet, Nutrition and Alternative Medicine is the autobiography of Marc Herlands, a young Jewish attorney who, beginning in 1974, at the age of twenty-six, had his career and personal life ruined by chronic exhaustion, severe pain, and terrible emotional and cognitive problems.

It took seventeen years before Dr. Gary Shima, MD began, in 1991, to discover the surprising causes of Marc's chronic illnesses and then apply many new techniques to heal him.

During the course of Marc's journey back to health, he learned many new techniques for healing chronic illnesses, such as obesity, alcoholism, chronic fatigue syndrome, fibromyalgia, Gulf War syndrome, rheumatoid arthritis, depression, chronic yeast and fungal infections, celiac disease, mycoplasma, heavy-metal toxicity / poisoning, and chronic viral infections.

During his long road to recovery, he also learned some valuable spiritual insights, which helped him cope with and endure his long-term illnesses.

He is especially grateful to Dr. Shima for finding the causes of his medical problems and discovering the remedies that cured his illnesses.

He is also especially grateful to Ms. Roxanne Watson, CHT, for helping him recover from his illnesses by applying her newly discovered techniques when using colon hydrotherapy.

Marc became chronically ill starting in November 1974. His symptoms came upon him suddenly at the age of twenty-six without warning and apparent cause.

His chronic fatigue and emotional distress left him unable to work full-time as an attorney during his first year in private practice.

By February 1976, his illnesses made it impossible for him to continue working as an attorney in Ohio, so he moved to Los Angeles seeking answers for his hypersensitivities to cold weather and limited amounts of sunlight, as well as his chronic fatigue and emotional turmoil.

In 1987, at the age of thirty-nine, while he was living in San Diego with his beloved wife, Louise, his life became unbearable.

In addition to his chronic exhaustion and depression, he began to suffer from severe pain throughout his body, especially in his legs. He had developed fibromyalgia.

That illness came upon him suddenly, without warning or apparent cause, exactly as his CFS had.

Two years later, in 1989, at the age of forty-one, Marc had become so exhausted that he was sleeping twenty hours per day.

He was in so much pain that he had to take barbiturates to make himself stay asleep. Otherwise, the pain in his legs would wake him every two hours, thus stopping him from getting any refreshing sleep.

Because of such frequent interruptions in his sleep, he was more tired when he awoke than when he went to bed the previous night.

In 1991, at the age of forty-three, after seventeen years of chronic exhaustion and four years of severe pain, suicide became a very attractive and reasonable option. In fact, Marc started to plan his final exit.

But in September 1991, Marc's luck changed for the better. Ms. Cathy Brady, a friend from law school, helped him find Dr. Morales, a dentist in Tijuana, Mexico, who specialized in removing mercury from old silver/mercury dental fillings. Removing those old fillings was the first relief from pain and suffering he had in over seventeen years. It was his first baby step back to health.

In November 1991, his wife found Dr. Gary J. Shima, a medical doctor in Encinitas, California, who specialized in the most challenging medical cases. His clinic specialized in caring for those patients where the causes of their illnesses were difficult to find and the remedies were unusual to prescribe.

In November 1991, Dr. Shima discovered that Marc had a *dysfunctional* immune system and *chronic* viral and bacterial infections.

In late 1992, through preliminary screening and standard medical testing, Dr. Shima found that Marc suffered from the *toxic effects* of *lead*, *mercury*, *nickel*, *vanadium*, and *cadmium* that had somehow accumulated in his body.

The sum of these parts was the beginning of a theory about why Marc had contracted CFS, fibromyalgia, and depression, and how to remedy those chronic illnesses.

About two years later, Dr. Shima found that Marc suffered from yeast and fungal infections and leaky gut syndrome.

Each of those illnesses played a significant role in causing his morbid obesity, confusion, depression, severe allergies, and internally produced alcoholism.

A couple of years later, Marc was diagnosed as having gluten sensitivity, or celiac disease. That condition (1) caused malnutrition due to not fully absorbing vitamins and nutrients, (2) stunted his growth, (3) prevented the elimination of toxic heavy metals from his body, (4) created severe constipation called impacted bowel syndrome, and (5) created constant fatigue and pain.

Dr. Shima also discovered that Marc suffered from a chronic unusual infection caused by *Mycoplasma fermentans incognitus.*

Mycoplasma is a highly dangerous, contagious, and debilitating pathogen. It was created by the US government as a biological weapon of mass destruction.

It was not designed to be immediately lethal, but it was designed to be totally exhausting and emotionally destructive. Luckily, Marc, with the help of Dr. Shima, was able to rid himself of this horrible bug twice.

Another piece to Marc's medical puzzle was added when he was diagnosed with a *neurological disorder* that caused him to have extreme fatigue, chronic pain, hypersensitivities to light, sound, and odors, and cognitive impairments relating to confusion, comprehension, and short-term memory loss.

Luckily, Marc responded well to medicines that reduced his symptoms caused by his neurological disorder. He has used Neurontin (gabapentin) to reduce his fatigue and pain; Lamictal (lamotrigine) to reduce his hypersensitivities to light, sound, and odors; and Diflucan (fluconazole) to reduce his cognition problems.

By 2002, at the age of fifty-four, after almost ten years of treatments and remedies (which included the use of medicines, antibiotics, oxygen, transfer factor, vitamins, minerals, herbs, amino acids, enzymes, essential fatty acids, chelation, colonics, acupuncture, chiropractic, lymph massage, diet changes, meditation, and removing the silver/ mercury fillings from his teeth), Marc's health had greatly improved—but not enough. He was still very tired and mentally challenged. His short-term memory and his vitality were still very limited.

But by 2013, after twenty-two years from the date of discovering the first of the major causes of Marc's illnesses, the exhaustion associated with chronic fatigue syndrome, the pain associated with fibromyalgia, the pain and despair associated with depression, the cognitive impairment associated with CFS and fibromyalgia, and his morbid obesity had disappeared.

After many decades of great pain and suffering, Marc feels he has fully recovered from his chronic illnesses and medical problems.

While he was on his road to recovery, he found there were many medical tests that could have been used to determine the underlying causes of his illnesses much earlier in his life if they had been ordered by his doctors. *There is a list of these tests in this book.*

If these tests had been performed when Marc's illnesses had begun, Marc may not have had to suffer so many decades of pain, exhaustion, and emotional and cognitive impairments.

During his twenty-two-year recovery period from 1991 to 2013, Marc found new techniques for healing that are not readily known to the public. Those techniques are both traditional and nontraditional, and many of them helped him recover from his illnesses.

Marc shares what has worked for him so that those who suffer from these illnesses may *suffer less* and *recover faster.*

Much of what Marc reveals is unusual or even controversial, but he believes that the final chapter on the causes of these illnesses and their ultimate cures has not yet been written.

Medical science has not yet provided definitive answers to these two important questions:

1. What causes CFS, fibromyalgia, obesity, and alcoholism?

2. Which remedies work best to alleviate the symptoms of those illnesses?

Marc believes that there is plenty of room for reasonable speculation and new ideas about (1) what causes those illnesses and (2) which treatments work best.

In response to those questions, Marc shares what he knows has worked for him using the insights and techniques provided by Dr. Shima, and what he believes will probably work for others.

Lastly, it is Marc's greatest wish that this book will spur doctors, healers, health-care practitioners, insurance companies, and government agencies into giving better care, better testing, and more financial support to this group of most unfortunate patients.

1

MY STORY: BIG CHALLENGES

I was born in 1948. As of March 2013, I was sixty-five years old. Those who do not suffer from any of the illnesses that cause brain fog (cognitive impairment) will not be impressed by my ability to do this math.

But those who do have cognition problems (and there are millions who do) will appreciate that I am able to do the math so easily.

There was a long period when I couldn't do the math very easily. That ability was taken away from me by my illnesses. Truly, I have come a long way.

If you have brain fog, you will know what I am talking about. Otherwise, you will not.

If you have brain fog—cognitive impairment or confusion—those neurological problems are sad, funny, cause anxiety and fear, and can be overwhelming. It is not pleasant.

If you have brain fog, you will understand how much I have suffered when I was not able to do arithmetic, remember simple tasks, or think straight. It was a profoundly, absurdly heart-wrenching three decades of my life.

You may have noticed that this book uses large print, wide margins, and extra space between paragraphs. This was done intentionally.

I did these things intentionally because I am writing for a group of people—*which includes me*—who have major difficulties reading, comprehending, and remembering what we have just read.

We must take extensive notes in the margins about what we have just read, or we will not be sure we have just read it.

We must write down our questions *immediately as they come to mind*, or we will forget them.

We need to underline as we read, or we will not remember what we have just read.

We need to make comments in the margin so we might have a small chance of understanding the material tomorrow.

We need to pause, think, ponder, and then think some more about what we read to try and grasp its meaning.

We need a lot of space in our books so we don't get confused.

I wrote this book using very simple language and easy-to-understand syntax. I wrote it this way because many of us have problems with cognition. Many of us do not understand complex sentences. We need written communication to be simple, direct, and straightforward, or we might not understand it.

I wrote this book for those who suffer from brain fog, or cognitive impairment. I did not write this book for those who do not.

Those of you who have brain fog will understand.

But those who *don't* have this problem, or *don't know* people who have this problem, most likely won't understand our challenges very well.

Those people won't understand because it is difficult to imagine how it feels when you just can't think straight.

I learned a lot about our illnesses when I was co-chair of the Chronic Fatigue and Fibromyalgia Resource and Support Group of San Diego, California.

I was co-chair for about five years in the late 1990s with Ms. Josephine Nost, who now lives near Tampa, Florida. She has been a wonderful friend of mine for a very long time.

Our group met monthly. We invited a professional in the field of CFS or fibromyalgia to speak to us. After the lecture, we socialized.

It was a loosely associated group of about four hundred people, most of whom were chronically ill from CFS or fibromyalgia. The others were caregivers for or supporters of persons with CFS or fibromyalgia.

I learned that as a group, we have *unique problems*.

First, I learned that our illnesses are basically *invisible* to the general public.

To the average person, we look healthy and well, especially when we are out in public, which is usually only for a brief period of time.

For the *average* person who is *disabled* with these illnesses, *we are only able to go out in public for an hour or two at a time.*

However, there are truly tragic cases. Some of the worst cases in our group included men, women, and young people who awoke, showered, and had to go right back to bed *because washing exhausted them for the day.*

People with our illnesses who get up, get washed, and get out for an hour or two look healthy *except if you look into our eyes.* It is then that you see the telltale sign of diminished vitality that is masked by our wan smiles and cheerful, uncomplaining countenance.

If you know what to look for, you will see that we are not well. But few people can see beyond our weak smiles and our decently groomed appearances.

Few people know how to look into our eyes and see beyond our tired smiles and weak voices.

As a result, our group *fools most people* into believing we are feeling better than we actually are.

Unless you had one of our illnesses, you wouldn't know that we were not well. But each member of our group would know because each one of us is always sick. Each of us is always tired.

Second, I learned from our group members that people who do not have our illnesses *do not understand* our suffering and despair.

I learned that all of us had, at one time or another, tried to explain to our family, spouses, friends, doctors, healers, and caregivers how we felt, what it meant to live with a chronic illness, and the horrible feeling of being always exhausted, continuously in pain, and in unremitting despair, hopelessness, and poverty.

I learned that all of us had, at one time or another, tried to tell our coworkers and bosses about our illnesses and medical problems in general terms.

But it was clear to me—from my own experiences and from listening to others—that unless you had our illnesses, you wouldn't understand what it feels like, and what it means to live every day feeling exhausted or in great pain.

When I was co-chair of the CFS and fibromyalgia support group in San Diego, almost everyone started their conversation with me with what it was like to live with their illness.

Each person started with

how *bad* they felt,
how *much pain* they were in,
how *tired* they were,
how *little* they could do,
how *badly* their *cognition* was,
how much physical, emotional, and financial *trouble* they
    were in, and
how *little understanding and support* they received at
    home from their spouse, family, and friends.

There were exceptions of course, but the general rule was *they were alone* in their despair, suffering, pain, and grief.

I learned that each member of that group carried on as best he or she could, but in general, very few of us received enough financial or emotional support from our family, spouse, or friends.

Hardly anyone received sufficient financial support from the government, a religious or local charity, their disability insurance company, their family, or generous friends.

Too often I heard how many of our members had been *abandoned* by their families, spouses, friends, bosses, and clergy because those people no longer had the strength to provide support. I learned that our members' illnesses wore out their family, spouse, friends, caretakers, clergy, bosses, and support system.

Even after telling them that they didn't have to tell me their stories because

I was one of them,
I knew what they were going through, and
I had all of the same health challenges they had,

they were so accustomed to being *misunderstood* by friends and family they felt *compelled* to tell me their stories and their complaints before moving on to their real interests, which were *always* the same:

1. What did my doctors find wrong with me?
2. What was I doing to get better?
3. Which doctors or healers could I recommend?
4. How could they get more money from the government or insurance company so they could pay their bills or go to more doctors?

Then our conversation really started.

They asked me their most pressing questions:

What had I learned about what might be causing our illnesses; how could they get better and recover?

As a result of

their continuous pain and exhaustion caused by their illnesses,

their overwhelming frustration caused by not knowing the causes of their illnesses,

their hopelessness caused by not being able to remedy their chronic health problems,

their depression caused by knowing they would never again be fully employed,

their despair caused by constantly living in poverty and destitution,

their continuing grief caused by having been abandoned by family, spouse, friends, the government, their community, and their insurance company,

too many members of our group had *suicidal thoughts,* and sometimes, someone actually *committed suicide.*

Sadly, a couple of good, decent, and loving members of our group took their lives because life had become *unbearable* for too long.

I have written this book for those who have been *left without answers* to their most basic questions about

the *causes* of their illnesses, and

the *remedies* that could work for them;

and for those who have been *left without hope* of /
   discovering the causes of their illnesses, or
   finding anything that might bring them some relief.

To those who have our illnesses, let me say this:
For decades, I was where you are now.

But by the grace of God, and for some unknown reason, my life has been spared, and I have recovered.

After decades of suffering, by luck, I stumbled upon a few doctors, dentists, and healers, who had *new ideas* about what caused my illnesses;

they had *new ideas* about how to fix me;

they were willing to risk the medical and dental establishments' challenges and use some *new* and *unconventional* techniques to heal me.

As a result, *I recovered.*

I hope and pray that this book may bring you much-needed relief as soon as possible on your journey to recovery.

Believe me, *my heart is with you, forever.*

2

Past Events, Future Problems

I realize that many of my various health problems arose from events that happened a long time ago. I can remember events that caused significant health problems much later in life.

From having interviewed hundreds of patients with CFS and fibromyalgia, I have seen that there are many similarities in our stories. I will use examples from my own life as a way of illustrating general principles that I believe to be true for most of us who have suffered from these illnesses.

Head and Neck Injuries

Many persons with CFS and fibromyalgia told me they had experienced *whiplash* injuries to their neck and head in the past.

They said that someone or something had *hit them* hard on the head or neck whereupon they blacked out or almost blacked out.

Some said they had experienced significant *falls* that had caused concussions, significant head injuries, head or neck traumas, or blackouts in the past.

I remember playing American football on the ice near Cleveland, Ohio, during the late fall and winter up until the age of eighteen. I played with six to twelve other big, strapping young men. None of us wore helmets or other protective gear. I remember banging my head on the frozen earth while being tackled and while tackling others. It was great fun then.

But looking back, my parents, teachers, doctors, and I were not very smart about the long-term health consequences that can be caused by having concussions and traumatic brain injuries. Now we are more aware of the long-term damages caused by traumatic brain injuries.

In the 1950s and 1960s, it was common for us kids to have "minor" head injuries that were caused by banging our heads on the ground when we tackled some guy or when we were tackled by the other guys. In those days, no one thought about the health consequences of having a concussion or any other type of brain injury.

Fast-forward fifty years to 2013. It is now recognized that traumatic brain injuries may cause significant health problems *years after the injury was sustained.*

But I believe it is still *unusual* for physicians, medical practitioners, and other healers to associate traumatic brain injuries with CFS and fibromyalgia. However, my research shows that there is likely causal relationship, but it has not yet been recognized in this field of medicine.

CELIAC DISEASE

Celiac disease is the inability of the body to properly digest wheat and other grains that contain the same gluten. It leads to an inflammatory condition throughout the GI tract. It is an autoimmune system disorder that affects the colon and small intestine.

It is now thought that celiac disease affects about 1 percent of the American population. It is believed that most people do not know that they have the disease since, many times, the symptoms are subtle.

I believe celiac disease played an important part in causing my severe exhaustion (CFS) and my severe pain (fibromyalgia).

Celiac disease can cause other problems as well. It can cause mild to severe *constipation*. In my case, when I was four years old, for the first time, I had severe abdominal pain. That was because I was severely constipated.

To alleviate my abdominal pain, my caregivers gave me an enema. It worked fine. But it should have been a *big tip-off* that I had a problem. My problem was that I could not digest wheat.

Unfortunately for me, that important piece of my health puzzle was missed by my doctors and healers for *more than five decades.* That was very bad for me. And it is very bad for people who have the illness and who are not properly diagnosed and given appropriate medical advice.

As a result of having celiac disease, I had abdominal pain. The pain was caused by having eaten white bread, which my body was not able to digest properly.

Because of celiac disease, the white bread became wadded up and *obstructed* my colon. That wad caused me to suffer *severe* abdominal pain.

Around the age of thirty-six, I suffered from such severe abdominal pain that I had to be admitted to the emergency room at a hospital in Washington, DC.

X-rays revealed that I had a large wad of undigested food lodged in my intestines. I believe the undigested mass was composed of undigested wheat and other grains containing the same type of gluten I could not digest. Again, celiac disease proved to be very painful for me.

Celiac disease can also be subtle. It can make you feel constantly weak, tired, and emotionally drained.

Celiac disease, I believe, can also wear out the villi in the intestines. Worn-down villi can prevent the body from absorbing sufficient nutrients, which can also make you feel weak, tired, and emotionally fragile.

In the extreme, celiac disease can also stunt a person's growth, as it did me.

When I was twelve, I stopped growing. After having been the second tallest boy in my class for years, I stopped growing and ended up being only average height.

When I was thirteen, I had extensive testing to find out why I had stopped growing. Unfortunately, my doctors did not discover the cause. They thought I had a dysfunctional pituitary gland. But I believe I had stopped growing because I had celiac disease.

If I had known in 1960 that I had celiac disease, I would have avoided eating wheat and other foods that contained the same bad gluten.

By avoiding wheat, I would not have suffered from most of the very severe health problems that affected me during my life.

If I had been told at the age of twelve that I had celiac disease, and I had been advised not to eat wheat and other foods that contained the offending gluten, most likely I would not have suffered a lifetime of such severe pain and chronic exhaustion.

But that diagnosis was missed for five decades, and celiac disease ended up causing me to have many big health problems in my life.

CHRONIC YEAST AND FUNGAL INFECTIONS

When I was twelve years old, I craved breads, cakes, ice cream, candy, and cookies. I was also continuously tired and hypersensitive to cold. Finally, I became fatter, rounder, and bloated.

These symptoms combined to create a pattern that should have been recognized by my doctors that I was probably suffering from chronic yeast and fungal infections.

COGNITIVE IMPAIRMENT

When I was twelve years old, I had my first episode of brain fog. Some call it "fibro fog" too.

Brain fog is the condition where you just can't think straight. It is a form of cognitive impairment.

You have brain fog when you go to the refrigerator, open the door, and cannot remember why you are there.

You have brain fog when you put your keys down, turn around, and can't remember where they are.

You have brain fog when you drive through a stop sign that you've stopped at a thousand times before because you didn't remember it was there.

You have brain fog when you have read the same paragraph ten times in a row and still can't remember what you have just read.

You have brain fog when you have read the same sentence ten times in a row and can't understand what you have just read.

Everyone does one of these things once in a while, especially when they are busy or distracted with some other thought.

But people with brain fog do these things almost every day—and sometimes many times a day, especially when they are not busy and have no other distractions or other thoughts.

BRAIN FOG HAS MANY CAUSES

Brain fog may be caused by a yeast or fungal infection that has spread throughout the body, up to and including the brain.

It may be caused by a mycoplasma infection.

It may be caused by heavy-metal toxicity, especially from lead.

It may be caused by a vitamin D3 deficiency.

It may be caused by a vitamin, mineral, amino acid, or enzyme deficiency.

It may be caused by hypothyroidism, adrenal exhaustion, hypoglycemia, or liver problems.

It may be caused by all of the above as it was in my case.

Emotional Problems

When I was fourteen, my emotions became hard to handle. I was tired and angry.

Obviously, adolescence played a large part, but there was more going on.

Yeast, fungus, and mycoplasma can cause those kinds of emotional problems.

In addition, when I was fourteen, I became a very chatty person. That was a sign I had *mercury toxicity*.

In the 1800s, English workers pounded mercury by hand into felt hats to make them pliable. Over time, mercury toxicity made the hat workers very chatty and compulsive talkers.

They were described as being "mad." Hence, the expressions "mad as a hatter" or "mad hatter" were created to describe those hatters who were affected by having absorbed too much mercury.

EMOTIONAL OUTBURSTS

When I was fifteen, my emotional levels were very high. I had a lot of anger. Emotional problems, especially anger, can be caused by an accumulation of heavy metals in the liver, a mycoplasma infection, yeast or fungus infections, alcoholism, malabsorption, or hypoglycemia. I am sure I had a lot of those things.

SHORT-TERM MEMORY DYSFUNCTION

When I was fifteen, my short-term memory became seriously problematic. It became much worse by the time I was sixteen.

At fifteen, I tried to memorize lines for a short school play. I rehearsed and practiced by repeating them many times. Even after repeating my part hundreds of times, I could not remember my lines.

By the time I was sixteen, my memory became much worse. I couldn't remember what I had been trying to memorize just a few minutes before. No matter how much I practiced, I could not make most things—anything—stick in my memory.

French class was my "Waterloo." (Pun intended.) I could not memorize French words and phrases or accomplish most of the language skills needed to succeed in learning a foreign language no matter how hard I tried.

DEPRESSION

By the time I was eighteen, I had my first episode of major depression. Thankfully, my case was fairly mild at that time. For the next few years until I was twenty-five, my depression came and went, and the symptoms were manageable, although the dark clouds of depression always seemed to threaten to make my life worse.

WEIGHT GAIN

From the ages of twenty-six until thirty-eight (1974 until 1986), I gained 116 pounds. I went from 130 to 246 pounds. I was five feet eight inches tall. I went from being skinny to morbidly obese.

After consulting over one hundred doctors, medical practitioners, and healers, no one could determine what caused me to be so ravenous and need to eat so much food.

In fact, I used to be hungrier *after I ate a meal* than before I started. Sometimes I ate two meals because I was still hungry after finishing the first one!

I now believe that my problem was caused by extreme yeast and fungus infections. I believe that when I started to eat, the yeast and fungus, which had spread throughout my body, became more active and demanded to be fed *more food*. Those entities are powerful monsters. I believe they made me eat much more than I personally desired, which caused me to gain a lot of weight.

CHRONIC EXHAUSTION

In 1974, at the age of twenty-six, my doctor said I was "burned out." He ordered me to rest more and work only part-time. He thought I was exhausted from working too hard, but that was not true.

I was working as a real estate and business attorney. My job consisted of preparing routine paperwork. It was not a very stressful or tiring job.

I worked seven hours per day and five days per week. A thirty-five-hour workweek was not very much for a first-year associate at a busy law firm.

In comparison, most first-year associates worked about seventy hours per week. My doctor and I did not know it then, but I was suffering from a full-blown case of CFS.

CFS

From the ages of twenty-six through forty-three (1974 through 1991), I was barely running on empty. I was totally exhausted. From 1987 to 1992, I was sleeping twenty hours per day. My day consisted of watching TV, reading a book, newspaper, or magazine, or grocery shopping. Even those few things made me exhausted after only ten minutes, and then I had to stop, rest, and even sleep.

FIBROMYALGIA

When I was thirty-nine years old (1987), I developed severe, chronic pain all over my body, but especially in my legs. It was horribly painful, especially at night.

I needed sedatives to make me sleep and stay asleep for at least six hours. Without the sedatives, the pain in my legs would awaken me every two hours, and I would not get a sufficient amount of good-quality sleep to feel even slightly rested. Without enough good-quality sleep, I was even more exhausted the next day.

DESPAIR

By 1991, at the age of forty-three, after seventeen years of chronic exhaustion and four years of severe fibromyalgia pain, I was in total despair.

I had no hope of recovering. I believed there were no remedies or cures for my health problems. I believed my health problems were only going to become worse. I was in total despair.

I had endured too much suffering and too much pain, and I had decided to find a way out of my misery. I was ready to end my suffering.

I remember setting a date—six months and two days in the future—which was the exact day my wife would be legally entitled to receive all the benefits from the life insurance policy we had purchased one and a half years before.

There was a suicide clause in that life insurance policy stating that after two years from the date of purchase, even if the insured commits suicide, the insurance company must pay all benefits to the surviving beneficiary. It cannot contest paying the benefits of the policy even if the insured commits suicide after two years from the date of purchase.

But if the insured commits suicide prior to two years from the date of purchase of the insurance policy, the company can choose to pay only the premiums collected, and it does not have to pay the amount promised in the policy.

I remember telling God that I had decided to wait until two years and two days from the date of purchasing the life insurance policy before I was going to commit suicide so that my wife would receive all the money from the insurance policy I had bought a year and a half before.

I had bought it so that my wife could pay off our mortgage just in case I passed away while we still owed money for our mortgage on our house. I remember telling Him that if He didn't want me to commit suicide, it was up to Him to fix me! I had tried everything I knew, and now I had put my fate directly into His hands.

Despite being married to the most wonderful, charming, beautiful woman on the planet, my despair had reached its limit. I had reached my breaking point. I had reached my limit. My pain and exhaustion had become too great for me to bear any longer.

Despite living in a wonderful new home in a very lovely city, despite having very good relationships with friends and family, I was without hope. I was in total despair.

By 1991, I was no longer able to work as a lawyer, even part-time, because I was too tired and too brain fogged to think straight. I could hardly remember any facts. My short-term memory had been destroyed.

By 1991, I was so tired that I could barely watch TV, read a book, listen to music, or go to the supermarket without falling asleep ten minutes later.

By 1991, I was sleeping twenty hours per day.

By 1991, I suffered from weird and strange afflictions.

Suddenly, without warning or cause, my hands swelled, doubled in size, and itched like crazy.

Suddenly, without warning or cause, my stomach bloated to twice its normal size.

Suddenly, without warning or cause, hives broke out over my stomach and abdomen.

At night, my legs had so much pain I had to take a sedative (Klonopin) to keep myself asleep for at least six hours. Otherwise, I would be awakened by the pain throughout the night and never get a full night's rest.

Each morning, I awoke more tired than when I went to sleep.

By 1991, I was living in misery. I was constantly exhausted, chronically in pain, always hungry, constantly angry, always confused, bitter, sad, depressed, and brain fogged. I was worn out.

By 1991, my only hope of escaping from my chronic pain and exhaustion was to commit suicide. Only the will of God kept me from completing that final act of obtaining relief.

But then, in early 1991, my luck changed. Dr. Morales removed the silver/mercury fillings from my teeth and replaced them with a plastic compound. For the first time in decades, I began to feel better.

However, by mid-1991, I relapsed. Then I met Dr. Shima. He diagnosed me as suffering from systemic viral infections and *immune system dysfunctions.* He ordered that I use transfer factor injections to help regulate and increase the effectiveness of my immune system.

Unfortunately, that treatment plan did not work well enough. But in late 1991, Dr. Shima found that I suffered from the toxic accumulation of heavy metals in my body.

He found that I had tremendous excesses of lead, nickel, mercury, cadmium, and vanadium in my tissues. I was literally storing a large amount of poison in my body, and I was literally poisoning myself all the time.

That diagnosis explained why I was so exhausted, in chronic pain, and so emotionally distraught for so many years. In late 1991, I began chelation treatments to remove the heavy metals.

When that was not successful, in early 1992, I began colon hydrotherapy (colonics) to do the same thing. After nine years of using colon hydrotherapy, that job was completed, and I felt much better.

However, a few years later, I was diagnosed with *celiac disease.*

That diagnosis explained why

1. I had *stopped growing* when I was twelve years old.
2. I was *constipated* throughout my lifetime.
3. I could *not properly digest and absorb* the nutrients from my food.
4. I could *not eliminate toxic heavy metals* from my body.

During the next two decades, other important diagnoses arose, which explained in more detail why I was so tired, in so much pain, and so emotionally distraught.

During that time, I was diagnosed with having

1. *Hypothyroidism*, which caused my constant fatigue and poor metabolic functioning
2. *Neuropathy*, which caused my fibromyalgia (pain)
3. *Hypersensitivity* to light, sound, and odors, which caused my exhaustion and pain
4. *Kidney disorder*, which caused my fibromyalgia (pain)
5. *Yeast and fungus infections*, which caused exhaustion, severe stomach bloating, obesity, *hypoglycemia,* brain fog, and balance problems
6. *Virus and bacterial infections*
7. *Flukes* (worms)
8. *Psoriasis*
9. *Depression*
10. *Neurological disorders*
11. *Mycoplasma fermentans incognitus* infection

It turns out that Mycoplasma fermentans incognitus was created as a biological weapon of mass destruction (WMD) by a scientist who worked for the US government.

Strangely, it appears that a patent has been issued to that scientist who was its creator.

It was created with the intention of making anyone who became infected with that WMD anemic and emotionally unstable.

Garth Nicolson, PhD, a medical researcher, has testified before Congress about this form of mycoplasma.

He has stated that he believes that this form of mycoplasma contaminated US soldiers during the first Gulf War and is most likely the *primary cause* of Gulf War syndrome (GWS). This finding is disputed by the US government. It is not that important as to whether this form of mycoplasma is the sole cause of GWS.

What is important is that if you think you suffer from GWS, you should be tested for this pathogen. If you have been infected by it, when cured, your life will be greatly improved.

Mycoplasma fermentans incognitus is a terrible pathogen. It *robs the body of energy*, and it causes chronic exhaustion.

It makes the body weak by invading the red blood cells, and then it destroys the cells' ability to use oxygen, iron, and vitamin B12.

Without oxygen, iron, and vitamin B12, I became chronically weak, tired, exhausted, anemic, and was in great pain.

When mycoplasma dies off, it creates major *emotional problems*. The die-off can cause severe bouts of anger to the point of rage and even violence. In addition, the die-off can cause severe pain (fibromyalgia).

For further information on treating mycoplasma, I have written in a later section of this book how I cured myself twice from mycoplasma infections using two different techniques.

During my journey back to health, I was diagnosed with other major illnesses as well. They included

1. Sleep apnea
2. Vitamin D3 deficiency
3. Enzyme deficiency
4. Adrenal exhaustion
5. Essential fatty acid deficiency
6. DHEA deficiency
7. Hypoglycemia
8. Syndrome X / Insulin insensitivity

Each of the above illnesses caused chronic exhaustion and brain fog.

It was a very long and exhausting process to discover the causes of my illnesses, and then to use various remedies to recover from them.

It took decades to discover the pieces of my medical puzzle, and then to put the pieces into a coherent order.

The interrelationship of these illnesses has *never been* explained in any textbook.

It turns out that *good testing and common sense* played a large part in discovering what was wrong with me.

Once the causes of my illnesses were known, the remedies were not too difficult to figure out.

However, many of the remedies had to be creatively utilized by my doctors, especially Dr. Shima.

This book is a compilation of what I learned from my doctors, health-care practitioners, healers, and other patients who had similar illnesses.

It is also a compilation of my own opinions, which are based upon my own experiences, the experiences of others, my reading and thinking about what I had learned from all my doctors, healers, and health practitioners.

During the thirty-nine years it took me to regain my health, I developed various theories about the causes of and remedies for my illnesses and some other chronic illnesses.

I hope that by sharing what I have learned, my experiences, my ideas, and my thoughts, those who suffer may find quicker, easier, and less expensive remedies for relief.

I hope those patients who suffer as I did will receive better care from their doctors, health-care providers, healers, caregivers, support system, friends, family, insurance company, and government.

To those who suffer from chronic illnesses,
I wish you the very *best* of luck.
I hope you *discover quickly*
the *causes* of your illnesses and
you *find* the very best *remedies very soon.*

3

Helping Others Improved My Health

When I was trying to find remedies for my illnesses, I often shared my knowledge with other patients and the many doctors, healers, and health-care practitioners who were helping me.

I found that the *more I willingly and generously shared* at my own expense, the *more remedies were revealed to me and the more I recovered.*

I discovered that the *more I gave* to others with a genuine wish to help those who were less fortunate, the *more* my health improved.

That was the *most* important lesson I learned when I was so ill.

As a result, I came to believe that the following sayings are true:

What goes around comes around.
As you do unto others, it will be done unto you.
The law of karma is beyond doubt.

Over the years, I have shared these lessons with many people.

So I take this opportunity to share them with you.

I place them first and foremost;
I consider them to be that important.

4

ACCEPTANCE AND TRUST IN THE HIGHER POWER

When I was very sick, I had the time and inclination to call upon God as my Higher Power for help.

I was helpless when confronted by my overwhelming illnesses.

I was left with only my faith in God and that my life was proceeding just as it should be—despite not going as I had previously planned.

I went from being the typical young American lawyer, who was full of himself and his self-assured future success, to completely surrendering to my fate that I was living with a situation where I was completely helpless.

I had no other choice in the matter because I literally could not do anything else. I couldn't read, watch TV, work, or play without falling asleep.

By 1991, my life had been reduced to eating, sleeping, and breathing. I could no longer work, play, or do productive things. I was that sick.

I lived day by day prayerfully, waiting and hoping that someday I might get well.

But in my time of total sickness, I was still able to help others—by listening to them, making suggestions, giving support, making them laugh, and taking care of my family's daily needs.

I came to realize that my future was no longer under my control because I was barely able to survive.

Over time, I accepted my fate and the fact that I had no control over my future.

I had to turn control of my life over to God. I could only wait for a miracle, or I was going to die.

I learned not to think about how I was going to make a living or control my destiny.

During those decades of great illness, I learned to surrender to the grace of God and believe that He had a reason for my becoming totally disabled.

I found it was good for my state of mind if I added a good amount of faith to my daily routine. That helped me get through the day.

It was comforting to me to believe that God had some kind of plan for my life even though his plan was not obvious to me.

Over time, I found myself becoming more compassionate toward those who were ill or less fortunate.

I could relate to them because I was now one with them. I could resonate with their lives and their stories because I too was one of the less fortunate.

I could see that my illnesses were making me a more compassionate person—even as they kept me from earning a lot of money, power, fame, and prestige.

I took comfort in my personal growth. I had no other choice.

It was nice to know that science had shown that prayer worked to heal people quicker.

But it felt better to know that I was getting closer to God as I lay sick on my bed, day after day, night after night.

Surrendering to my fate brought me peace of mind, especially as I endured great pain, exhaustion, and suffering.

I found that it was best if I stopped worrying about the future and put my faith in God.

I found wonderment and even some joy in my life's journey—even if this was not the kind of life I had planned when I was a young attorney with great ambitions.

After a few years, I accepted my new reality. I surrendered to the idea that I was no longer going to be an attorney who was going to have great fame and fortune.

Instead, I saw myself as a person who was destined to become more compassionate and who had a lot of unusual but useful health information to share with doctors, healers, and those in need.

I became fascinated by my transformation from attorney to healer. I found happiness when I accepted my fate, my destiny, and my karma.

Being ill, I realized, was my life's adventure. Every day, I was on a very dangerous adventure trying to find what ailed me, and then trying to find a cure.

It was a fascinating journey because every day brought a surprise of finding that my doctors had discovered that I suffered from a new illness.

My life became my own personal drama, which was also fascinating.

At all times, I knew that the end of my adventure might result in my death—I was that sick.

Or the adventure might somehow lead me to recovery.

I had no idea how my drama was going to end. All I knew was that with God, all things were possible. And only He could save me.

I began to take each day as it came—one day at a time, one step at a time. I had no hope, but I had gone beyond total despair.

Without hope, I waited daily for God to work His miracles on me. I prayed. And I went on day by day.

My life became my own personal drama. I became the main character in my own story of life and death. Interestingly, I did not know how the story would end.

In the context of my life being a life-and-death struggle for survival, my story became very interesting to me.

Each day, a new piece of information was added to my health puzzle. Patterns were starting to be revealed.

Almost daily, my doctors revealed new discoveries about my illnesses. That process gave me hope and interest. I had passed beyond the time of my great despair.

> **I** came to understand that God was the playwright of my drama.

> **I** came to know that my life was completely and totally in His hands.

> **I** came to know that I would live or die based only on what He ordained for me.

I watched myself go through my illnesses as an audience watched a play, except I was the main character in my own drama. And I was the audience as well.

Since I had no idea of how my drama would end, it was very interesting and really very dramatic to me.

I came to know that no matter how much I wanted to know the conclusion of my life's drama, it was not going to be revealed until God decided it was time for me to know that information.

I came to understand these truths:

1. Life is on a "need to know" basis.
2. When God wanted me to know something, He will reveal it.
3. Life moves on God's schedule.
4. The truth will *not* be revealed before its time.

I stopped demanding that God reveal the end of my drama to me. I stopped asking Him when or if I would recover. Instead, I relaxed and let Him run my life.

I tried to remember that my health issues were just another episode in my life's drama.

I tried to find enjoyment in each day's events, no matter how painful or exhausting.

I realized that to stay happy, I had to stop worrying about the future.

I realized that worrying about my health would not change the present, past, or future.

I realized that I should not worry about the future because it would not make me feel better. It would only make me feel worse.

So I tried to limit worrying when, if, or how my drama would end.

I realized that I should give up getting upset about not being able to pursue my prior goals as an attorney and businessman. That was the past. That was not what he wanted me to do.

I tried to relax and took one day at a time.

I surrendered to my fate.

I surrendered to the fact that my life was literally in God's hands.

I surrendered control of my life to Him. He was the Absolute Captain of my ship.

That meant if He wanted me to get better, *He* had to do it. My life was under His control.

That also meant if He didn't want me to get better, I wouldn't.

It was up to Him to heal me. If I were to get better, it would be on His terms, on His schedule, and in His way.

Because I was at wit's end, over time, I surrendered to my fate of being totally disabled, and I made peace with the Lord.

As I forced myself to change my point of view from being an egocentric, materialistic Western man to a spiritually centered, surrendered-unto-God, yogi man, a few very interesting things began to happen.

Insights came to me which seemed profoundly important.

One insight was that I had to go through these illnesses in order to gain these insights.

Another insight was that it was my calling to be sick so that I could learn and understand some very basic spiritual truths.

Over time, deeper spiritual truths became apparent to me.

I began to understand that to reach my highest happiness, it was necessary to make my heart fill with love and compassion at all times.

I began to understand that I was here to serve God and to serve others in love, peace, and harmony.

I began to understand that
each of us is here on planet Earth to learn

to love God and to love each other.

I began to learn that

love is caring and sharing.

Falling in love is a *bio-karmic* electromagnetic attraction.

I laughed. I realized that prior to my illnesses, I had heard those words but had not understood their meaning.

As I lay chronically exhausted and in severe pain day after day, year after year, those words became living testaments that resonated in my heart and soul.

I laughed at what pain and suffering it took to make me realize their more significant meaning.

I began to understand that we humans grow wiser through suffering.

This was a truth that became very apparent to me over time.

I laughed at how simple those truths were.

I began to understand that we humans grow more mature by "taking up our individual crosses" and by sacrificing pleasure for the sake of spiritual gain.

I began to learn that irony and paradox were the touchstones of truth.

I began to learn that the books of Job and Genesis were very important to me.

I began to realize that those insights would not have come if I had been healthy and worked as a businessman or an attorney.

I began to realize that my illnesses had given me the time and opportunity to commune with God.

I began to realize that He had given me the time and opportunity to commune with Him.

I began to realize that my illnesses had given me the chance to enter into the Spirit of God.

I began to realize that my illnesses had given me the time and opportunity to discover what I needed to know about the meaning of life.

We are all angels-in-training,
and planet Earth is the *boot camp* for the soul.

I began to realize that those insights had given me great peace of mind, humor, fun, joy, love, compassion, and a desire to be of greater service to others despite my body being very sick and not being very successful financially.

I began to realize that during my illnesses, God had the time to work His magic on me and He was *transforming* me into a *wiser* and *more compassionate*, *humane* human being.

I considered that a fair trade. I took on a sick body in exchange for an improved heart and soul.

I began to think that my illnesses were a blessing in disguise.

I began to realize that my illnesses had

refined my soul,

allowed me to purify my thoughts,

permitted me to enter the kingdom of heaven in
order to receive greater understanding,

made me a much better, more compassionate,
happier person.

I began to realize that having those kinds of insights made
me very happy.

I began to be happy that my life turned out the way it had,
illnesses and all.

I began to realize that I still struggled with my desire for
more money.

I began to realize that taming the inner demon is part of
the process of becoming more humane.

For all of the above, I have become grateful and happy
despite having experienced the physical, mental, and
emotional crucibles of suffering for a long period of time.

I began to see that my illnesses helped me grow wiser,
more loving, and more compassionate.

I began to see that when I was young, becoming a more humane person was not something I thought was of much value.

I began to see that becoming a more *humane person* was the only thing of value, and becoming a more *humane person* was the only thing worth striving for.

I began to see how we humans are deluded into pursuing false gods.

It's funny that I didn't see all these things when I was well. I only realized these truths when I had been ill for a very long time.

I began to think that all of the above was amazing.

My heart began to be constantly filled with joy because God had replaced the old, selfish me with a more loving and compassionate me.

I found myself thinking this:

> When I am in my that place of love, and
> you are that place of love,
> then we are truly blessed and are one.

Namaste.

5

Chronic Fatigue Syndrome (CFS) Has No Medically Defined Cause or Causes

Chronic fatigue syndrome (CFS) is just what it says it is. It is a syndrome. Therefore, there are no specific underlying causes for the illness.

However, I found from my own experience and from speaking with others that there are many similar causes of the chronic fatigue syndrome. I discuss them in this book.

The chronic fatigue syndrome is a *descriptive* diagnosis. It is a diagnosis that is reached by the doctor only after he or she has *excluded from possibility through testing and diagnosis* every other illness that looks like CFS.

There are certain characteristics of CFS, but they are not causes. If the patient's illness has those characteristics, but his or her doctor cannot find any specific cause for the chronic exhaustion and other symptoms, then the doctor gives the patient a diagnosis of chronic fatigue syndrome.

For example, after testing reveals that the patient does *not* suffer from things like lupus, cancer, herpes, mycoplasma, hypothyroidism, heart disease, HIV, Epstein-Barr virus, sleep apnea, mercury toxicity, or depression, the doctor will diagnose the patient as suffering from CFS.

If the patient is told by the doctor that he or she has CFS, it means that the patient suffers from chronic exhaustion and a few other symptoms, but he or she does not know the cause. That is the reason CFS is called a syndrome and not a disease.

Being diagnosed with CFS tells the patient only what he or she *doesn't* have. That may be comforting, but it does *not* tell the patient what he or she *does* have. That is a big problem for the patient.

If the patient *doesn't know* what is causing his or her chronic exhaustion, it is very difficult—or almost impossible—to find a cure or an appropriate remedy.

Without an accurate diagnosis of the cause of chronic fatigue syndrome, the doctor is shooting in the dark if he or she attempts to prescribe an appropriate remedy. In that situation, the likelihood of a successful resolution of the patient's case is moderate at best.

The longer people have chronic fatigue syndrome, the more likely that the cause and remedy will never be found, and the patient will suffer indefinitely.

6

CHRONIC FATIGUE SYNDROME IS NOT DEPRESSION

CFS looks like chronic depression, but it is not. There are major *differences* that distinguish the two disorders.

There are many *similarities* between CFS and chronic depression. Both types of patients are without much energy, stay at home very often, and don't seem to be able to do much.

Someone can have CFS and depression at the same time. They are *not mutually exclusive* illnesses.

However, there are some very important *differences* between a person with CFS and one who has chronic depression.

First, CFS patients generally *do not react favorably to antidepressant medications* unless they suffer from depression as well.

Often, patients with CFS report very bad side effects from taking antidepressant medications. This does not generally occur with people suffering from depression.

Bad side effects occur with CFS patients because CFS is *not* a serotonin problem.

Second, CFS patients most often *cannot tolerate exercise* without becoming seriously ill. The bad side effects from exercise may last a day, many days, or even a couple of weeks.

On the other hand, patients suffering from *chronic depression* generally report that exercise *helps* them feel much better.

Quite often, a patient who suffers from depression will swear that his or her exercise program is medically necessary to maintain his or her physical and mental health. Patients who suffer from CFS do not find that exercise improves their mental health or moods at all.

CFS patients do *not* get a "runner's high." We wonder,

"Why do other people enjoy exercise so much?"

because it is *not* an enjoyable part of our life's experience (if it ever was).

When CFS patients exercise too much, we often become very ill. That is radically different from patients who suffer from chronic depression.

Third, CFS and fibromyalgia patients *actively seek out advice* from many doctors and healers when we are searching for causes, cures, and remedies.

We actively search the Internet for the latest developments about our illnesses.

We read magazines and newspaper articles about our illnesses. We join groups to discuss our illnesses with others who have our problems.

We are very proactive when trying to recover until we become overwhelmed physically, emotionally, or financially.

Then we become reclusive because we no longer have enough energy or other resources to keep going.

Patients with CFS and fibromyalgia *actively search* for many different kinds of doctors and health-care professionals from a variety of sources while patients with chronic depression do this much less.

Patients with CFS and fibromyalgia go to *many* health-food stores, health conventions, and alternative healers while patients with chronic depression do this much less.

Patients with CFS and fibromyalgia use the opinions of *many* doctors, healers, and health-care practitioners and will try many different kinds of remedies while patients with chronic depression will seek out the opinion of just one or two doctors, take just one or two pills, and if that does not work, will do nothing more.

Patients who suffer from CFS and fibromyalgia tend to be *proactive* in their recovery process while those who suffer from chronic depression do much less. I exaggerate to make these points.

Fourth, chronic depression may be caused by excessive amounts of *cortisol*. Medications may help reduce excessive amounts of cortisol and relieve that kind of depression.

CFS is *not* caused by excessive amounts of cortisol, so those kinds of medications do not eliminate CFS *unless* CFS is also caused by yeast and fungus infections—then there may be an overlap of those illnesses. Some medications may alleviate both sets of problems.

Many doctors are not aware of some of these differences. It is an area of medicine where doctors may need to use more caution to avoid causing additional harm to CFS and fibromyalgia patients.

7

CHRONIC FATIGUE SYNDROME IS HEAVY-METAL TOXICITY

After seventeen years of disabling exhaustion, I was diagnosed with suffering from the toxic effects of heavy-metal accumulation. I suffered from excessive amounts of mercury, lead, nickel, vanadium, and cadmium that were stored in my body.

Each of these heavy metals is very toxic, very poisonous, and all of them had accumulated far in excess of the maximum safe level.

After seventeen years of becoming progressively worse, Dr. Shima and his assistants discovered that I was being poisoned on a daily basis by those heavy metals.

The basic effects from heavy-metal poisoning were as follows:

disabling exhaustion

chronic confusion

brain fog

severe pain

emotional disorders

hypersensitivities to sound, light, and odors

unrestful sleep

post-exercise dysfunction

malabsorption

digestion and elimination dysfunction

immune system dysfunction

yeast and fungal infections

viral and bacterial infections

mycoplasma infection

endocrine system dysfunction

Dr. Shima performed *three preliminary medical tests* to determine if I had heavy-metal toxicity.

First, I had a hair test;

Second, I had a live blood-cell analysis;

Third, I had an electrodermal prescreening test, which is an electronic wave machine test called the Interro—which analyzed by computer, my body's responses to the various electrical impulses that were sent through the electrodes I held in my hands.

Each of these preliminary tests accurately identified that I had high levels of heavy metals in my body.

Finally, after the preliminary testing, Dr. Shima performed a *standard medical test* using a *chelating* agent to determine the precise level of heavy metals in my body.

That standardized test conclusively proved I was suffering from the toxic effects of *excessive amounts of lead, nickel, mercury, vanadium, and cadmium*—all heavy metals, which had accumulated to excessively large amounts in my body.

ABSORBING AND STORING

Questions:

1. *Where* did I get those heavy metals?
2. *Why* did I store them?

Answers:

1. I *absorbed* the heavy metals from the environment.
2. Since my colon was clogged from the effects of **celiac disease**, I *stored* these heavy metals.
3. I stored them because it was *too dangerous* for my body to discharge them from my liver into my colon because they would end up in my bloodstream, thus poisoning my body and brain.

I absorbed heavy metals
from the environment.

When I was growing up from 1948 to 1969, there were no significant environmental regulations. It was a time in the United States before there was the federal Clean Air Act and the Clean Water Act.

I absorbed mercury **from the environment.**

I absorbed mercury from the fillings that were used to fill the cavities in my teeth. I absorbed mercury when I polished dimes with it when I was a child. I absorbed mercury when I used Mercurochrome to disinfect cuts I had suffered as I played as a child.

I absorbed mercury by breathing mercury-contaminated fumes emitted from the coal-burning electric power plants in my city.

I absorbed lead from the environment.

Lead was in the paint that was on the wooden slats that kept me safe in my crib as an infant. I teethed on those wooden slats, ate the paint, and absorbed the lead.

Lead was in the paint that coated the No. 2 orange pencils that I used in elementary school. I chewed on those pencils, ate the paint, and absorbed the lead.

Lead was in the tap water. It leached into the water from the solder that was used to weld the copper water pipes together.

Lead was in gasoline—which I breathed and absorbed.

I loved breathing those gasoline fumes. I *loved* inhaling those fumes because my body was substituting the oil in the gasoline fumes for essential fatty acids that were deficient in my diet and body.

My body was making that substitution in order to stay alive and grow. It was a short-term fix, but it caused long-term problems.

I absorbed nickel **from the environment.**

Nickel was in my stainless-steel cookware, my stainless-steel cutlery, and in my stainless-steel braces that were on my teeth for six years.

Nickel was in my French horn's stainless-steel mouthpiece, which I played almost every day for six years.

I absorbed vanadium **and** cadmium **from the environment.**

Vanadium was in our air. I breathed it and absorbed it. It came from the steel mills that were upwind. It came from our electric power plant that was upwind.

I absorbed cadmium from cigarette smoke. It was absorbed firsthand when I smoked a little, and I absorbed it secondhand when my parents smoked in my presence.

Absorbers vs. Excreters

I breathed and ate those heavy metals, and my body did *not excrete* them well enough to keep me healthy.

Instead, my cells and organs *absorbed* them. As a result, over time, I became very sick from absorbing too many heavy metals. Unfortunately, I was an *absorber*.

Everyone breathes and eats some heavy metals from the environment, but their bodies do not absorb them very much. Instead, their bodies excrete them. They are *excreters*. As a result of excreting most toxins, most people do not suffer the problems I did.

Because I had celiac disease, I believe that my body did not excrete those heavy metals. Instead, my body *stored and absorbed* them. The result was I became very sick with CFS, fibromyalgia, and depression.

After seventeen years of being chronically ill, constantly exhausted and in pain, without any diagnosis, I was without hope of recovery. My total despair made me suicidal.

Without hope, I saw no point in living. Suicide had become a settled issue in my mind.

I literally challenged God saying, "If You don't want me to come home, it's up to You to fix me."

Surprisingly, He did!

Obviously, He had other plans for me, and He wasn't about to let me commit suicide.

Let me finish this section by sharing one of my favorite, ironic, and humorous bits of truth.

"If you want to make God laugh, tell Him *your* plans!"

I told Him my plans when I told Him I was going to commit suicide—and He laughed.

Over the next twenty-two years, He caused me to recover my health—very slowly and with great effort. But recover I did.

Looking back, my plan to end my suffering in six months and two days didn't work out. In fact, *no plans in my life* worked out.

But I see now that I'm much happier because none of them worked out!

Go figure!

I have learned from life's experiences that *irony and paradox rule.*

8

CHELATION AND COLONICS SAVED MY LIFE

After Dr. Shima determined I was suffering from the toxic effects of having accumulated excessive amounts of heavy metals in my body, the obvious course of action was to remove the heavy metals.

He recommended that I start on a program of using chelating agents to remove the heavy metals. In late 1991, at the age of forty-three, I began to use chelation.

Chelation is a medical procedure where a chemical agent is put into a body through a vein in the arm by a slow, intravenous drip over a three-or four-hour period.

The chemical then binds with the heavy metals as well as all other electrically charged particles in the body.

The body then excretes the heavy metals and all other electrically charged particles, called *electrolytes,* during urination.

There is a potential problem with chelation. When the electrolytes are removed, the electrical system of the body, including the brain and nerves, are put at risk from depletion. Over time, the body may suffer harm.

To avoid potential problems, electrolytes in the form of minerals are put back into the body by using an IV drip.

In fact, I had three IVs per week. Two were chelations, and one was an electrolyte replacement.

After the first six weeks, I had twelve chelations and six electrolyte replacements. I felt great. I thought my doctor had found *the* cure. However, that was not to be true.

After the ninth week, I had eighteen chelations and nine electrolyte replacements, but my body had become too weak and exhausted to continue.

Dr. Shima was mystified. He did not understand what was going wrong. So we decided to stop the chelation treatment.

He recommended that I use colon hydrotherapy (*colonics*) to flush out the heavy metals from my body.

In late January 1992 at the age of forty-three, I had my first colonic.

I was amazed because it worked so well.

From the first colonic, I felt great relief. I was amazed because my body did not suffer any bad side effects as I had experienced with chelations. Most importantly, I felt great afterward.

Because I had felt such great relief from the first colonic, I decided to continue.

After each colonic, I felt wonderful. In addition, there were no negative side effects. The proof of the pudding. Colonics made me feel better.

During each colonic, I could *see* and *feel* toxins leave my body.

I felt the toxic load in my body being reduced *during and after* each colonic. I knew that the level of poisons in my body was going down, and *I was going to recover.*

During and after each colonic, I felt I was witnessing a miracle. I watched my vitality and life slowly return to me in health, joy, and happiness.

I was constantly filled with awe, happiness, and gratitude during those amazing years that I gratefully shared with my wife.

During each colonic I literally *felt* the toxins leave my body. Whenever the toxins were released from my body, I felt the stress. I used to break into a sweat and became light-headed from the toxic release.

Also, I *saw* the water—which passed out of my body and then through the tube on the colonic machine—*change color*.

I saw the water turn from clear to *neon yellow* when the heavy metal toxins were released from my body. Sometimes I saw the water turn from clear to *bright pink* when lead was released from my body.

My recovery detox process was very slow.

During the first two years, I had three colonics per week.

For years 3 and 4, I did two colonics per week.

For years 5 and 6, I did one colonic per week.

For years 7 and 8, I did one colonic every two weeks.

It took almost nine years for my body to release all the toxins I had accumulated during my lifetime. It was a very long, slow, laborious process.

I learned to honor my body's time schedule of release and recovery. I could not do it faster, or I would have hurt myself. I had to become a very *patient* patient (pun intended) to regain my health.

Since the ninth year, I have one colonic every four or five weeks because I have a body that accumulates toxins.

Because I take many medicines for various unrelated health issues, they can cause an accumulation of toxins during the month.

I continue to use colonics on a monthly basis to remove the accumulation of those toxins in order to continue feeling great.

Since 1992, Ms. Roxanne Watson has been my colon hydrotherapist. Words cannot express how I feel about her. I owe her so much gratitude for helping me heal and keeping me on my road to recovery during the past twenty-two years.

9

THE COLONIC PROCESS

In a nutshell, the colonic can be described as follows:

The colon hydrotherapist infused my colon with water and stimulated my liver to dump its stored toxins into the water. The toxin-filled water was deposited into my colon and was then removed from my colon through the use of the hydrotherapist's colonic machine.

To help stimulate my liver, the hydrotherapist used her hand or a vibrating machine to pump moderately on my abdomen just above my liver while I was filled with water during the colonic.

That palpitation stimulated my body to release toxins into the water, which were then dumped into my colon. My colon then dumped the toxic-filled water out of my body, and it passed through the colon hydrotherapist's colonic machine.

After the wastewater left my body, I could see it passing through the tube that was on the colonic machine.

Most often, as water left my body and passed through the machine, the water was clear, or it carried some limited amount of waste material. At that point, it was not filled with toxic materials.

However, when my body dumped toxins into the water, the water changed color. The water often went from clear to *neon yellow*. Sometimes, it went from clear to *neon red*.

As the toxins left my body, I felt the effects of the release. It caused sweating and sometimes a little light-headedness for half a minute or so, but those symptoms passed quickly.

But the benefits I had from the colonic were so great that the minor side effects were soon forgotten. After the colonic, I felt great. Feeling so good made me want to do it again.

Soon after the first few colonics, the process became repetitive. It seemed that during the next couple of days, more toxins were released by the cells in my body, and those toxins were then moved and stored in my liver, waiting to be released during the next colonic.

The next colonic caused my body to again release newly stored toxins into the water. The toxin-filled water was again dumped out of my body through my colon. The toxic water passed through the colonic machine where I watched it move through the clear tube, which was part of the colonic machine.

After nine years of religiously using colonics, my body released almost all toxins and heavy metals that had accumulated during my lifetime.

As the amount of toxins in my body lessened, I slowly regained my health.

Colonics, indeed, *saved my life.*

10

COLONIC DISCOVERIES

During the process, Dr. Shima, my colon hydrotherapist, and I made some startling discoveries.

1. When I used *ultrasound* on my liver or teeth during a colonic, it *greatly increased* peristalsis. I called this a *sonic colonic*.

2. When I used various colored lights—but especially *blue light* emitted from a low-powered cool laser, or *infrared light*—on the liver or teeth during a colonic, it greatly increased peristalsis. I called this a *photonic colonic*.

Peristalsis is the muscular process by which the body moves food in the throat through the stomach, the small and large intestines, and finally, removes solid waste from the body.

3. When I used ultrasound or light on any part of my abdomen or teeth during a colonic, it greatly increased the amount of *waste matter* I released during my colonic.

4. When I used ultrasound or light on any part of my abdomen or teeth during a colonic, it greatly increased the amount of *toxins* and *heavy metals* and *lymph material* I released during my colonic.

5. My body *dumped toxins from my lymph system* during a colonic.

11

SIGNS OF LYMPH DRAINAGE

First, lymph material was seen going through the clear glass tube on the colonic machine. It looked like bits and pieces of wispy mucus.

Second, when the lymph material was released from my body, I experienced severe sweating.

Third, when the lymph system discharged its toxins, there was a fair amount of pain. The pain was much worse than that which occurred when the body released its toxins. However, the sweating and pain lasted no more than a minute or two.

Fourth, when the lymph-release stopped, all of the above symptoms stopped, and *I felt wonderful.*

Because of the great health benefits I received from colonics, I lovingly share my motto with you:

A clean colon is a happy colon!

12

More Benefits from Colonics

1. *Colonics promote beautiful skin.* When toxins are removed from the body, which may have accumulated from smoking cigarettes, the skin appears clear, radiant, and youthful into old age.

Think of the film and stage actress Mae West and her beautiful skin. It is my understanding that she used colonics regularly.

The skin is the fourth largest organ of detoxification in the body after the intestines, lungs, and lymph system. When toxins have been removed from the body, the skin is relieved from processing their removal and is under much less stress. The result is more beautiful-looking skin.

2. *Colonics promote weight loss and size reduction.* When I removed excess waste matter from my body, I lost weight and reduced my size.

When toxins and poisons were removed from my body, my cells retained less fluid and shrank in size and volume. The result was I lost weight and reduced in size.

My food metabolism and assimilation were improved through the use of colonics. I required less food to maintain my energy and vitality. The result was I lost weight and reduced in size.

3. *Colonics can reduce lower back pain.* When excess waste matter accumulates in the colon, the nerves in the lower back can be chronically stimulated. That can lead to lower back pain. When excess waste matter is removed through colonics, lower back pain can be reduced.

4. *Colonics promote lymph-system drainage and cleaning.* Colonics help stimulate the body to remove waste matter from the lymph system. Colonics also clear the colon so the body can safely discharge this highly toxic waste matter from the lymph system.

The lymph system is the *garbage dump* of the body for toxic waste. The lymph system surrounds each of the cells, and the cells dump their waste into the lymph system. The lymph system is very large. It has three times the volume of the blood supply. When my lymph system became full of toxins, I became exhausted.

A lymph system is difficult to clean. Colonics are one method of promoting the expulsion of toxic material from the lymph system.

There are other ways to *stimulate the lymph system* to help rid itself of toxins and waste matter.

Some methods are

- Vigorous marching
- Pumping your arms and legs up and down
- Jumping up and down on a trampoline
- Jumping up and down without a trampoline
- Vigorously massaging the lymph nodes
- Using light on lymph nodes

13

CHRONIC FATIGUE SYNDROME HAS MANY CAUSES

CFS has many causes. The following is a list of many of them:

1. CFS is yeast or fungus overgrowth or die-off.
2. CFS is immune system dysfunction.
3. CFS is a weak immune system.
4. CFS is leaky gut syndrome.
5. CFS is allergies.
6. CFS is vitamin deficiencies or imbalances.
7. CFS is mineral deficiencies or imbalances.
8. CFS is amino acid deficiencies or imbalances.
9. CFS is enzyme deficiencies or imbalances.
10. CFS is Sjögren's syndrome.
11. CFS is essential fatty acid deficiencies or imbalances.
12. CFS is celiac disease.
13. CFS is malnutrition.
14. CFS is slow brain functioning.

15. CFS is fast brain functioning.

16. CFS is hypersensitivity to light.

17. CFS is hypersensitivity to sound.

18. CFS is hypersensitivity to odor.

19. CFS is dysrhythmia between breathing and heart rate.

20. CFS is pointed-head syndrome.

21. CFS is a mycoplasma infection
    (*Mycoplasma fermentans incognitus*).

22. CFS is flukes.

23. CFS is Epstein-Barr virus.

24. CFS is cytomegalic virus.

25. CFS is herpes virus.

26. CFS is post-polio malaise.

27. CFS is thyroid dysfunction.

28. CFS is sleep apnea.

29. CFS is hypothyroidism.

30. CFS is pituitary dysfunction.

31. CFS is hypothalamus dysfunction.

32. CFS is adrenal exhaustion.

33. CFS is kidney dysfunction.

34. CFS is liver toxicity.

35. CFS is mitochondria dysfunction.

36. CFS is hypoglycemia.

37. CFS is insulin resistance.

38. CFS is diabetes.

39. CFS is whiplash injury.

40. CFS is slipped disc.

41. CFS is pinched nerve.
42. CFS is emotional trauma.
43. CFS is post-traumatic stress disorder.
44. CFS is spiritual trauma.
45. CFS is attention deficit disorder.
46. CFS is attention deficit hyperactivity disorder.
47. CFS is not lupus.
48. CFS is not Lyme disease.
49. CFS is not anything else.
50. CFS is fibromyalgia but with much less pain.

These are probably the most important things I believe that cause CFS. I say this after interviewing hundreds of people with CFS and from my own personal experience.

I have spoken with hundreds of patients at various clinics I have attended, as well as so many of the four hundred members of the Chronic Fatigue Syndrome and Fibromyalgia Research and Support Group of San Diego, California, which Ms. Jo Nost and I co-chaired for about five years in the late 1990s. Most of our members had CFS or fibromyalgia, but a few were supporters and caregivers of people who had this illness.

Obviously, my conversations were not scientific, but I believe that they gave me a broad general understanding about

CFS, and about the commonalities that seemed to appear quite frequently as causes of this illness.

The list was compiled from listening to all those people and speaking to many doctors and healers who had treated many patients with CFS. After a while a cluster of common causes seemed to emerge.

14

FIBROMYALGIA IS THE SAME AS CFS BUT WITH LESS FATIGUE

After listening to hundreds of people with CFS and fibromyalgia, I have seen and heard how similar these two illnesses are. I consider fibromyalgia to be the sister illness of CFS.

People with fibromyalgia have many of the same symptoms and problems as people with CFS, but they have less or little fatigue or exhaustion. CFS emphasizes the fatigue and exhaustion while fibromyalgia emphasizes the pain.

15

Fibromyalgia: A Kidney Disorder

Dr. R. Paul St. Amand, an endocrinologist in Marina Del Rey, Los Angeles, California, believes that almost all fibromyalgia patients have a kidney disorder, which creates plaque (calcium phosphate) in the cells—and that plaque causes severe pain throughout the body.

Dr. St. Amand's remedy is to use large doses of guaifenesin.

Unfortunately, that medication caused me to have excessive constipation, so he prescribed the medication sulfinpyrazone, which is now available for purchase only by prescription from Canada.

His contribution to saving the lives of many people with fibromyalgia cannot be overestimated.

My life has been greatly improved because of his medical discovery. For those so inclined, I suggest viewing his website for more information.

I had a huge success using his protocol, and I thank him immensely for his contributions to this field of medicine because, during much of my life, the plaque caused my muscles to be hard as rock.

But to be honest, I have known many others who have not been as fortunate as I. For those who have not responded well to his protocol or will not respond well, I have found there are other causes of and remedies for fibromyalgia, which I list and discuss next in this book.

16

Fibromyalgia Has Other Causes

1. Flukes: infection and die-off
2. Yeast and fungus: infection and die-off
3. Mycoplasma: infection and die-off
4. Lyme disease
5. DHEA problems
6. Adrenal exhaustion
7. Post-polio syndrome
8. Hypoglycemia
9. Lymph-system toxicity
10. Heavy-metal toxicity
11. Leaky gut syndrome
12. Sleep apnea
13. Vitamin D deficiency
14. Vitamin B deficiencies
15. Mineral imbalances and deficiencies
16. Amino acid imbalances and deficiencies
17. Essential fatty acid imbalances and deficiencies

18. Bad mattresses
19. Whiplash
20. Pinched nerves
21. Pointed-head syndrome
22. Damaged tendons and ligaments
23. Toxic muscles
24. Damaged cartilage
25. Stored or repressed negative emotions
26. Post-traumatic stress disorder

17

PROLOTHERAPY HELPS FIBROMYALGIA POINTS OF PAIN

Prolotherapy is the injection of a benign substance into the ligaments and tendons to repair irritated and chronically injured tissue. The website *Prolotherapy.com* states that:

> Prolotherapy is also known as nonsurgical ligament reconstruction. Prolotherapy uses a dextrose (sugar water) solution, which is injected into the ligament or tendon where it attaches to the bone. This causes a localized inflammation in these weak areas, which then increases the blood supply and flow of nutrients, and stimulates the tissue to repair itself.

Dr. Shima used prolotherapy injections on many of my fibromyalgia points of pain during the course of my recovery. I found that each treatment gave long-lasting relief in those areas of acute pain.

18

CHASING AND POPPING FIBROMYALGIA POINTS OF PAIN

I discovered a technique that slowly reduced my fibromyalgia points of pain. Literally, I had thousands of them.

When I was lying on the couch or bed, I closed my eyes and located the worst fibromyalgia point of pain in my body.

Then, I did the following *technique*:

1. I squeezed my muscles until I found the most painful fibro point of pain in my body.
2. I zeroed in on that specific fibro point of pain.
3. I relaxed all other muscles in my body.
4. I squeezed the fibro point of pain as hard as I could for as long as I could.
5. I rested.

6. I repeated.

7. I located the next most painful fibro point of pain in my body.

8. I zeroed in on that one.

9. I relaxed all other muscles.

10. I squeezed the muscle with that fibro point of pain as hard as I could for as long as I could.

11. I rested.

12. I repeated *until there were no more fibro points of pain or until my time ran out or until I became too exhausted to continue.*

13. I knew I had reached the "most important fibro point of pain" when I had squeezed it for as long as I could, and then I began to *fibrillate.*

14. The **fibrillation** lasted a few minutes.

19

Repressed or Suppressed Memories Can Cause Fibro Points of Pain

My fibro points of pain were located in the knots in my muscles. Some of the knots were created by tensions that had started when I was very young.

Sometimes when I fibrillated, a flashback or memory of some tension-filled incident with some person would come to mind.

I realized that one cause of a fibro point of pain was the tension stored in the core in the knot in the muscle.

I realized that the muscle knotted into a ball of pain because there was a very specific incident of tension.

I realized that the muscle stayed knotted in a ball of pain because the memory was stored in the tension-filled muscle.

I realized that when I squeezed that last worst fibro point of pain as hard as I could for as long as I could, and then fibrillated, the flashback appeared in my memory and then disappeared.

At the same time, the knot in my muscle and the fibro point of pain dissolved and disappeared. Both were gone forever.

I realized that this flashback of memory and the dissolution and disappearance process of the knot in my muscle and the fibro point of pain occurred only when I fibrillated.

Each time it happened, it was a very exhausting process, but it left me exhilarated. *It also left me with much less pain.*

Popping and dissolving the fibro points of pain was a very fascinating, exhilarating, long-term process.

Over time, I removed over 99.9 percent of the fibro points of pain from my body.

I am very happy not to have them anymore.

20

Chasing and Popping Fibro Points of Pain: The Technique in Plain English

I started by lying down in a comfortable position, usually on my bed, and then I closed my eyes.

I started by squeezing all my muscles and discovered which *fibro point of pain* was the worst.

I squeezed the muscle that contained the *worst* fibro point of pain. I squeezed that muscle as hard as I could for as long as I could.

Then, I gradually focused on the specific fibro point of pain.

I squeezed that fibro point of pain as hard as I could for as long as I could.

Then I rested.

Then I repeated.

I would find and locate the next worst fibro point of pain and repeat the process.

I literally chased the fibro points of pain around my body for an hour or two each day.

After an hour or two, there came a time when there was no worst fibro point of pain.

After I squeezed the last worst fibro point of pain for the day, as hard as I could for as long as I could, I began to **fibrillate**.

My body shook for a minute or two.

Then I knew I had popped a major center of tension and pain. Many times, a repressed memory or flashback popped up.

If that happened, it was an image of a person with whom I had had some previous tension.

I knew that the tension had been stored in a knot in my muscle, and it was causing a fibro point of pain.

By squeezing that fibro point of pain as hard as I could for as long as I could, I released the memory that was causing the muscle to stay knotted.

After that knot was released, that fibro point of pain was released too, and both disappeared forever.

I have used this technique for more than three years. It has eliminated over 99.9 percent of my fibro points of pain.

I am now virtually free from fibro points of pain.

Hallelujah!

In Conclusion

For those who wish to know my present status, at almost sixty-five years of age, I am left with some minor pains, which appear if I work or exercise too hard, become too stressed out, or when the weather changes.

The level of pain that I now have is *hardly noticeable* compared to the level of pain I lived with for decades.

To say the least, *I am one very happy camper!*

21

Medical Cannabis (Marijuana) May Reduce or Eliminate CFS and Fibromyalgia Pain

When I have exercised too much, worked too hard, have felt too much stress, or when the weather changes, I feel some residual CFS exhaustion or some minor residual fibromyalgia pain.

I found that a little good-quality medical cannabis (marijuana) reduces or eliminates my residual CFS and fibromyalgia as well as some minor depression. A good sativa elevates my mood and makes me happy!

For occasional pain, I have used a little gabapentin (Neurontin) or an over-the-counter pain reliever.

I find exercise of no value for relieving my CFS or fibromyalgia. In fact, exercise makes my pain worse if I do it more than I can safely handle.

The amount of exercise I can tolerate varies. It depends upon my mood, the level of my vitality, the level of my physical strength, and my inner joy.

I do not exercise beyond my capabilities because *if I do too much, I will suffer* a significant *increase* in *pain* and *exhaustion* for a period of time.

Obviously, an increase in those negative side effects is not good and is to be avoided.

22

Silver / Mercury Fillings Can Cause CFS and Fibromyalgia

The fillings in my teeth were made mostly of *silver* and *mercury*. The mercury in those fillings caused the following:

1. Yeast and fungus overgrowth, which caused
2. Leaky gut syndrome, which caused
3. Allergies, hives, and psoriasis,
4. CFS, fibromyalgia, depression, brain fog, confusion, central nervous system dysfunction, balance problems.

For almost a century in the United States, dental fillings were made by mixing a few metals together according the following general formula.

25 percent silver,

50 percent mercury,

12 percent zinc, and

3 percent of a few other metals

One of my medical consultants, Dr. William Kellas, has poked ironic fun at the American Dental Establishment by saying:

> When *mercury* arrives at the dentist's office, it comes in a container that is clearly marked "Poison."

> And when mercury is removed from a patient's mouth, the dentist places it into a container that is clearly marked "Poison."

> *But* while mercury is in a patient's mouth, dentists tell patients that "those fillings are safe and harmless." How absurd!

It is *not acceptable* for anyone to say that fillings containing mercury are safe and harmless.

23

METHYL MERCURY GAS CAN CAUSE CFS

In addition, *methyl mercury gas* can be produced when someone chews food while they have a silver or mercury filling in their mouth.

Sometimes, the level of methyl mercury in a person's mouth can be over a thousand times *greater* than what is legally permitted to be in the environment by the US government.

It is obvious that some people are poisoning themselves into sickness or early death by the methyl mercury gas that is in their mouths.

However, we, the people, are *not* informed by our doctors or dentists of this toxic gas or its harmful effects.

It is not unreasonable to believe that many people with CFS, fibromyalgia, and other disorders have become very sick and died from the toxic effects of having silver or mercury fillings put into their mouths.

If they had been informed about the toxicity of silver or mercury fillings, many people would have been spared much misery.

The *good* news is that for most people, it appears that when mercury breaks off from a filling, it is excreted by the body without causing too much harm.

Also, it appears that for most people, they do not suffer too much from methyl mercury toxicity.

The *bad* news is that many CFS patients and fibromyalgia patients are absorbers of heavy metals, including mercury, and we are *badly affected by mercury* and *methyl mercury gas.*

24

MERCURY CAN CAUSE LEAKY GUT SYNDROME

Mercury acts as an antibiotic. It kills both good and bad bacteria. When it kills good bacteria in the colon, yeast can grow beyond its normal, healthy limit. Then yeast is able to change into fungus, and yeast and fungus multiply into the danger zone.

Fungus is very dangerous because it is able to drill holes through the walls of the colon and then enter into the bloodstream. It literally creates holes in the colon.

Holes in the colon allow yeast, fungus, pathogens, and unnatural proteins to pass into the bloodstream from the colon. Those things were supposed to stay in the colon and not get into the bloodstream.

When yeast, fungus, pathogens, or unnatural proteins enter the bloodstream, each can trigger the immune system to react a lot. A severe immune system reaction can cause the patient to experience mild to severe allergy attacks, hives, psoriasis, autoimmune disorders, or feel like he or she is always experiencing the flu or a chronic infection.

When a patient experiences the discomfort, pain, fatigue, and suffering of having holes in his or her colon or of having unnatural things pass through them, he or she is said to be suffering from leaky gut syndrome.

In addition, while in the bloodstream, yeast and fungus are being attacked by the immune system. Their death causes *die-off*. Die-off can cause severe reactions. Die-off can cause mild to severe allergic reactions, hives, psoriasis, fatigue, exhaustion, cognition problems, and mild to severe abdominal bloating. These are also symptoms of the leaky gut syndrome.

Yeast and fungal infections in the bloodstream may affect the brain. If the brain is affected, the patient can suffer various mental and physical illnesses, including depression, cognitive challenges, confusion, brain fog, short-term memory loss, and balance problems.

Please note that because the above illnesses were caused by yeast and fungal infections that affected my brain, medications such as Diflucan (fluconazole) and Sporanox have helped me (and others) recover from these problems.

Leaky gut syndrome may be remedied by using *butyric acid*. Butyric acid is a component of butter and ghee. It helps the body close the holes created by fungus.

Once the holes are repaired, the yeast, fungus, and other pathogens and proteins will no longer be able to reach the bloodstream, and the symptoms of leaky gut syndrome will diminish or subside completely.

Afterward, glutathione, yeast and fungal killers, and probiotics may be used to help reduce and heal the problems associated with leaky gut syndrome.

25

LEAD CAN CAUSE CFS AND FIBROMYALGIA

Lead is a very toxic heavy metal. It has been proven that it can cause major neurological disorders, especially in children.

Lead poisoning leaves you feeling very tired, exhausted, mentally dull and achy. It causes CFS and fibromyalgia.

The US government has a policy of wanting to prevent people, especially children, from developing severe neurological disorders caused by consuming lead-based paint or breathing lead-based gasoline.

Because lead is so dangerous, the US government ordered automobile manufacturing companies to stop producing cars that use leaded gasoline and produce automobiles that use unleaded gasoline.

Because lead is so damaging to the brain, the US government ordered gasoline manufacturers and paint makers to remove it from production in 1979.

Unfortunately for me, I stored large amounts of lead. As a result, I ended up with significant neurological disorders that caused extreme exhaustion, memory problems, and cognition and balance difficulties.

I believe that because I had celiac disease, my body stored lead instead of excreting it.

For decades on a daily basis, unknown to me, I was being poisoned by lead and other heavy metals *until I* removed them by using colonics.

26

EXPOSURE TO LEAD IN THE ENVIRONMENT

Instances where I was exposed to and ingested lead include the following:

1. I ate the paint off the No. 2 orange pencils I used in elementary school.
2. I inhaled leaded gasoline fumes.
3. I drank tap water that contained lead.
   Lead was leached into the water from the solder that was used to weld the copper water pipes together.
4. I ate lead-based paint that was on the slats of my baby crib.
5. I inhaled firsthand and secondhand cigarette smoke.

27

REGULATION OF HEAVY METALS IS GOOD FOR BUSINESS

Environmental regulation is necessary for personal safety, but it is also very good for business.

When you consider how many *millions* of people are *disabled* partially or fully, mentally or physically because they suffer from heavy-metal poisoning, lost productivity and payments to the disabled make the costs of heavy-metal toxicity staggering.

Protecting people from heavy-metal poisoning is not just doing good for people, but it is also *doing good for business.*

28

A Badly Functioning Immune System Can Cause CFS and Fibromyalgia

When the immune system is very active, you feel very sick and tired. You feel like you have the flu.

If you have leaky gut syndrome, chronic infections, or chronic parasite infestations, your immune system will be very active all the time. Then you will feel very sick and tired *all the time*.

The immune system stays active when it is trying to kill the invading bugs, but it is not able to kill all of them. It must stay active in order to stop them from growing, proliferating, and eventually killing your body.

When the immune system has sufficient numbers of white blood cells to fight the bugs but the white blood cells are not strong enough to kill the bugs, the immune system stays active all the time.

When the immune system stays active continuously, as when you have a cold or the flu, you will feel sick and tired, exhausted, and have aches and pain—*all the time.*

When that happens, life will become very grim.

If that happens, you may become chronically depressed.

29

A Dysfunctional Part of the Immune System Can Cause CFS and Fibromyalgia

When you do not have a certain part of your immune system, the bugs, germs, and pathogens can multiply.

You will feel sick and tired when the bugs take over your body.

You will feel sick and tired when they emit a lot of their waste.

You will feel sick and tired when they die off.

There are many different parts to the immune system. If any of the parts are not functioning well or are missing, your body may not be able to rid itself of the invading germs. If that happens, you will feel sick and tired and in pain *all the time*.

There are immune system specialists who have tests to determine the state of your immune system.

There are medicines to improve and repair a dysfunctional immune system.

It is important to know that CFS and fibromyalgia can be caused by one or more problems with one or more parts of your immune system.

30

CELIAC DISEASE AND MALNUTRITION CAN CAUSE CFS

Celiac disease has been diagnosed in about 1 percent of the US population. That means about 3.3 million people in the United States have the disease.

Millions of Americans should not be eating wheat, oats, rye or barley, and products containing those grains.

Eating those grains causes problems—both large and small—for people who have celiac disease.

Earlier, I wrote about how celiac disease affected my life:

1. I suffered severe constipation starting when I was a young child.
2. It had stunted my growth as an older child.

3. It blocked elimination as an adult, which forced me to go to the emergency room for treatment of my severe abdominal pain.
4. It led to my body storing heavy metals until I was poisoned by them.
5. It made me suicidal.

Celiac disease also caused me to suffer severe malabsorption. It prevented my body from absorbing enough nutrients causing severe fatigue and exhaustion (CFS).

When I did not absorb sufficient nutrients such as vitamin D3, I felt very tired to the point of feeling exhausted and kind of suicidal.

To *increase my energy*, I have used one or all of the following separately or together as needed:

50 mg vitamin B complex
general amino acid complex
vitamin D3 capsules
NADH

To better *digest and absorb nutrients* from my food, I use a general herbal enzyme supplement.

31

CELIAC DISEASE AND A LOW-CARBOHYDRATE DIET

Eating a low-carbohydrate diet to lose weight may work for some people because they have celiac disease.

If someone has celiac disease and *stops* eating wheat and other grains that contain the harmful gluten, their body will stop retaining fluids and start eliminating more waste and fluids.

As a result, they will lose weight and reduce in size.

I think this is a reasonable explanation simply because it happened to me.

32

Slow Brain-Functioning Can Cause CFS and Fibromyalgia

Many people have had brain injuries from whiplash or concussions. Those traumas may have *slowed* the functioning of their brains so that their brains are partially asleep despite the fact that they are awake.

They feel like they are tired all the time, mentally sluggish, and confused. Memory problems are triggered by slow brain-functioning too.

Fibromyalgia may be caused by slow brain-functioning as well.

33

FAST BRAIN-FUNCTIONING CAN CAUSE CFS AND FIBROMYALGIA

Many people have had brain injuries from whiplash or concussions. These traumas may have *increased* the functioning of their brains so their brains do not rest while asleep. This can lead to total exhaustion. They are tired and in pain all the time. I have used Neurontin (gabapentin) to help resolve this problem.

Beware, gabapentin can become a trap. I have known a few people who started using this medicine but had trouble stopping it when it was not effective or it was no longer effective.

Considering the challenges some people have had with this medicine, it is probably best to use the *lowest dose possible* because it can become great trouble if you have to stop using it.

34

Hypersensitivity to Light May Cause CFS

Those who are hypersensitive to light may become very tired. Eyedrops may help alleviate this problem.

35

Hypersensitivity to Sound and Odor May Cause CFS

Excessive hypersensitivity to sounds or odors may cause or be caused by CFS or fibromyalgia.

Sometimes, hypersensitivity to sound and odor may be caused by low vitality of the immune system or mitochondria.

To increase my body's vitality, I have increased the intake of vitamins, minerals, amino acids, essential fatty acids, and enzymes.

I have also increased the amount of time I am exposed to sunshine, and the length of time doing mild physical exercises, gentle breathing exercises, and meditation.

Reducing stress through yoga, laughter, and singing may also be helpful.

I have used Lamictal (lamotrigine) to reduce my hypersensitivities to light, sound, and odors.

Excessive light, sound, and odors can cause allergic reactions.

Benadryl and other anti-allergy medications may be beneficial for stopping allergic reactions caused by light, sound, and odors.

36

Dysrhythmia between Breathing and the Heart Rate May Cause CFS

One graduate student in psychology, whose name has escaped me, has researched the relationship between the breathing rate and the heart rate of CFS patients.

He told me the preliminary results showed that in healthy individuals, the breathing rate and heart rate were synchronized. But in CFS patients, this was not true.

The theory is too new to evaluate, but it could be something to think about in the future.

37

POINTED-HEAD SYNDROME MAY CAUSE CFS AND FIBROMYALGIA

Some babies come from the womb with the top bones of their head forming a ridge. If not corrected, these bones will continue to grow that way into adulthood, and they will form a pointed ridge down the top of the head on the adult. Since the ridge is covered over with hair, it generally goes unnoticed later in life.

However, some healers believe that having a bony head ridge has negative effects on health that can lead to CFS or fibromyalgia.

The theory is that if the bones are interlocked, they will not expand and contract as intended while breathing. Failure to do so may lead to toxicity, fatigue, and pain because the spinal-cerebral pump is not fully activated.

It is something to consider because I have been told by some healers that some people have had great relief by removing the pointed ridge on their heads through therapy (not surgery).

Personally, I have used constant head, neck, and trapezius-muscle massage to detoxify the muscles holding the bones in place.

Once the muscles were detoxified, I used moderate force to push on the cranial bones to gently nudge them into their normal positions.

As a result, I ended up with a completely round skull after having a pointed head for almost forty-eight years.

It took about three years from the time I was forty-eight to fifty-one years old, but now I have a round head without a pointy ridge running down the center of my skull.

38

FLUKES CAN CAUSE CFS AND FIBROMYALGIA

Flukes are flatworms that may come from eating meat. They are parasites that can cause fatigue and pain, CFS and fibromyalgia.

39

Epstein-Barr Virus Can Cause CFS and Fibromyalgia

EBV is a herpes virus. If it is not suppressed by the immune system, it can cause continuous exhaustion. If not totally suppressed by the immune system, it can cause unremitting activation of the immune system. An overactive immune system can cause CFS and fibromyalgia.

EBV is contagious, usually transmitted by kissing. It is commonly known as mononucleosis.

It is not considered a primary cause of CFS or fibromyalgia because people recover from it on a regular basis, and it is its own disease.

40

Cytomegalic Virus Can Cause CFS and Fibromyalgia

Cytomegalic virus, if not suppressed by the immune system, can cause continuous exhaustion and pain, thus causing CFS and fibromyalgia.

Like any other constant viral infection that is not remedied or suppressed, the virus may cause CFS and fibromyalgia.

As discussed before, a constantly activated immune system, which is trying to destroy the CMV, can cause CFS and fibromyalgia.

41

HERPES VIRUSES CAN CAUSE CFS AND FIBROMYALGIA

There are many herpes viruses. If any are not suppressed by the immune system, they can cause continuous exhaustion and pain. They may cause unremitting activation of the immune system. That, too, can cause CFS and fibromyalgia.

42

Post-Polio Malaise and Adrenal Exhaustion Can Cause CFS and Fibromyalgia

CFS and fibromyalgia patients who exercise too much may suffer exhaustion for days or weeks afterward.

CFS exhaustion is similar to what polio victims suffer after they exercise too much. That condition is called post-polio malaise.

For CFS and fibromyalgia patients, I believe that *adrenal exhaustion* and *DHEA deficiency* problems play large roles, especially when there are significant post-exercise malaise problems.

43

Sleep Apnea Can Cause CFS and Fibromyalgia

Sleep apnea is a neurological disorder that prevents patients from getting sleep that fully rejuvenates the body, mind, and spirit.

As a result of not getting fully rejuvenating sleep, patients suffer chronic exhaustion such as those who suffer from CFS and fibromyalgia.

You can have sleep apnea, CFS, and fibromyalgia together. They are not mutually exclusive.

44

Hypothyroidism Can Cause CFS, Fibromyalgia, Confusion, and Depression

Hypothyroidism is a medical condition where the thyroid gland is not performing well. As a result, the body's internal temperature is cold. The hair is brittle and lusterless. The patient will feel sluggish and depressed too. Aches and pains are felt as well.

Doctors do not treat borderline hypothyroidism because they generally do not believe that a cold body is too important. They are taught to believe that a hot body, one that has a fever, is in danger from infection or disease, and thus is in need of immediate treatment.

They are taught that a cold body is not in great danger of dying or becoming very ill very soon, so that problem is not in urgent need of treatment.

Nevertheless, it is a *big* problem for those of us who live in bodies that are chronically underperforming.

For example, think of an automobile. It is designed to work best at a certain temperature. If it is constantly running cold, the mechanic will try to discover what is wrong and fix the problem in order to *maximize performance*.

However, doctors do not think like mechanics. They are more worried about life-threatening illnesses to be overly concerned about people who are struggling through the day because their bodies are underperforming.

However, it is very important to have an internal body temperature that is within the normal functioning range. Otherwise, all other bodily systems will *not* function well either.

The normal internal temperature for optimal functioning is around 98.6 degrees Fahrenheit.

If you *feel cold* or have other symptoms of hypothyroidism, you may be a candidate for treatment. You may respond very well to supplemental treatments.

Lastly, for those who suffer from cold feet at night, I found that I had to *bundle up* to cure my cold feet!

I use a shirt, an undershirt, and a hoodie to keep my upper body and head warm. When I keep my upper body and head warm, my lower body, feet, and toes stay very nice and warm too.

All of this helps me sleep better at night. I wake up feeling more refreshed, relaxed, and happier.

45

Gulf War Syndrome and Mycoplasma fermentans incognitus

Mycoplasma fermentans incognitus causes CFS, fibromyalgia, depression, rage, and may be the *primary* cause of Gulf War syndrome.

Mycoplasma is its own kind of bug. It's a pathogen that is sort of like yeast and sort of like bacteria.

If you become infected by mycoplasma, it is very hard to get rid of. It is very contagious. It can be given to animals as well. It causes fatigue, exhaustion, pain, confusion, memory problems, rage, anger, and brain fog.

Mycoplasma fermentans incognitus is a very specific type of mycoplasma that is even harder to get rid of than normal.

It was created and *patented* (No. 5,242,820) as a biological weapon of mass destruction by a scientist working for the US government. It was created as a vehicle for *warfare*. It was created to infect the enemy and cause total disability but not death.

It was meant to debilitate many soldiers, support staff, and civilians—but not kill them. It was meant to cause the enemy to use huge amounts of manpower, energy, and supplies to take care of their sick, and thus hinder their ability to wage war effectively.

It was thought to be the *primary cause* of the Gulf War syndrome by Garth Nicolson, PhD, who has testified to this fact before Congress.

46

How I Killed Mycoplasma

I have had two major infections of mycoplasma in the past twenty years. It is unknown whether it grew back after a decade's relapse or I contracted it a second time from another source.

Here are the two different ways I killed it.

A. To kill mycoplasma recently (in 2012), I used *colloidal silver* injections three times a week for eight months to a year.

B. To kill *Mycoplasma fermentans incognitus* more than ten years ago, I used a combination of therapies.

First, I saturated my body with oxygen at ten liters of pressure for two hours, twice per day, by breathing it through a face mask.

I did this because oxygen weakens this parasite.

I believe that using a hyperbaric chamber to saturate the body with oxygen would also work well to weaken this parasite.

Second, I used the antibiotic doxycycline.

Third, I used an immune-system booster called a *transfer factor*, which was prepared by Said Youdim, PhD, of Los Angeles, California.

Fourth, I used an anti-allergy substance prepared at the clinic owned by Dr. William Ray in Dallas, Texas.

Fifth, I used my mind to create an environment that was inhospitable to the parasite.

Every day, I said to myself that my body was too hot for the mycoplasma to live in, and it had to go.

I thought of the following example:

When I think I am sucking on a lemon, my body reacts as if I am actually sucking on a lemon.

I realized if I thought that my body was too hot for the parasite to survive in, it will become too hot for the mycoplasma to survive in. Thus, it will have to leave or die.

Every day, I told my body to make it impossible for the mycoplasma to live in.

Every day, I told my body that the mycoplasma had to leave.

Every day, I told the mycoplasma it had to go.

Sixth, I put a low-grade electrical current on my body to change my body's electrical frequency. This made my body's electrical frequency inhospitable to the mycoplasma.

The electricity generator was sold by Dr. Hulda Clark of San Diego, California. Now the company is called Clarkia.

Seventh, I prayed and had others pray for me.

Eighth, ozone therapy may also destroy mycoplasma.

47

OBESITY AND TOXICITY

When I first removed the heavy metals by using colonics, I lost a lot of weight and reduced in size quickly and easily.

I believe that *my fat cells stored the heavy metals* because my body was not able to safely dispose of them during normal bowel movements or when urinating.

When my fat cells were storing the heavy metals, dieting did not work for me. Once the heavy metals were being safely removed from my fat cells, I was able to lose a lot of weight and reduce in size quickly.

As the heavy metals were being removed, I lost about forty pounds. I went from 245 to 205 pounds, and I have maintained that weight for more than fifteen years.

48

Obesity and Essential Fatty Acids

Olive oil, flaxseed oil, borage seed oil, fish oil, CLA, and evening primrose oil may be necessary in various amounts for some people to balance their diets and stop binge eating.

Each oil contains different properties. Some may reduce depression, which may be a cause of binge eating.

I found evening primrose oil, which is well-known for reducing mood disorders, including *premenstrual syndrome,* to be an effective mood elevator for me. It seems to help *relieve* my depression.

However, it did not help me lose weight. But it may help some people.

49

OBESITY MAY BE CAUSED BY YEAST AND FUNGUS

I have observed that when I was suffering from too much yeast and fungus in my body, I became bloated and heavier. But when I took Diflucan or Sporanox for a few days, I became less bloated and lost weight.

Why? Did my fat cells retain fluids as a defense against being invaded by yeast and fungus? Did my cells retain fluids to ward off the yeast and fungus invading them?

I do not know the answers to these questions. However, it is interesting to note that whenever I stopped eating *sugar*, *bread*, or *starch*, and I stopped drinking *alcohol*—all the things that yeast and fungus love—I did not become bloated, and I lost weight.

Others have reported the same thing to me, so I am sure there must be a *connection* between yeast, fungus, bloating, and obesity.

50

OBESITY AND YEAST: A CONNECTION

Yeast loves sugar, bread, starch, and alcohol.

Once yeast starts to feed on these things, it grows and demands more.

Once it grows and enters the bloodstream, it eats the sugar that was meant to nourish the brain.

Since sugar is the primary source of energy for the brain, not enough sugar in the bloodstream is a major problem for the body and brain. Without enough sugar, the brain will not work very well, and the body will become jittery and faint. That is the essence of *hypoglycemia*.

The brain demands sugar to function. It demands to be fed very fast. Otherwise, it and the body will not survive.

Without enough sugar, you feel jittery, faint, aggressive, or exhausted. These symptoms are known as having the "sugar blues."

When we need sugar fast, we reach for sugar, bread, starch, or alcohol. Each of these things are converted into sugar and can be used by the brain very fast.

This process floods the bloodstream with sugar and feeds the brain. *It also feeds the yeast.* And this process also makes us fatter.

As we feed the brain, we feed the yeast. The brain is fed but so is the yeast. The more we feed the brain, the more the yeast grows.

As the yeast grows, it demands more food. It eats the sugar that the brain needs. Thus, the brain is deprived of the sugar it needs. The brain screams for more sugar. We get the sugar blues. We feed it sugar. We feed the brain. We feed the yeast. This process is known as *hypoglycemia.*

And as we eat more sugar, bread, starch, and alcohol, we grow fatter.

Because of yeast, we eat too much of things like ice cream, potato chips, french fries, ketchup, and drink too much soda pop and alcohol. Literally, as we feed our brains, we grow our yeast.

Yum for us, and yum for our yeast—as we grow *more obese.*

51

ALCOHOLISM MAY BE CAUSED BY YEAST AND FUNGUS

Yeast loves sugar, bread, starch, and *alcohol*. Once yeast starts to feed on these items, it grows and demands more.

Once yeast enters the bloodstream, it eats the sugar that was meant to feed the brain.

Since sugar is the primary source of energy for the brain, the lack of sugar in the bloodstream is a major problem for the brain. When there is too little sugar in the bloodstream, the brain demands to be fed more sugar—fast.

As a result, we feed the brain sugar, bread, starch, or alcohol, all of which are converted into sugar for the brain very fast.

This process floods the bloodstream with sugar, which feeds the brain, but it feeds the yeast and fungus as well.

The result is that your brain is happy, the yeast and fungus are happy, and we grow fatter.

When we feed the brain, we feed the yeast and fungus.

The brain is fed, but so are the yeast and fungus. *The more we feed the brain, the more the yeast and fungus grow.*

This is a vicious cycle. This is the yeast monster.

As the yeast grows, it demands more sugar, bread, starch, or alcohol.

Some people's brains crave alcohol. If that happens, they suffer from *alcoholism*.

The more alcohol they drink, the more they feed their yeast and fungus.

As their yeast and fungus grow, they deprive their brains of sugar.

Then their brains demand that they feed it more alcohol.

Repeat.

Hence, they become *alcoholics*.

Drink alcohol!

Yum for them, and yum for their yeast and fungus.

At an Alcoholics Anonymous meeting, the participants eat lots of doughnuts and cookies and drink coffee with lots of sugar and milk.

It seems clear that alcoholics are *substituting* sugar, bread, and starch for alcohol. They do this to *feed their yeast.*

In my opinion, if alcoholics would *reduce* their yeast and fungus, they would be able to *reduce their alcoholism* as well.

From my observations, this makes perfectly good sense to me.

52

FSF AND CFS, FIBROMYALGIA, CONFUSION, AND DEPRESSION

Foul-smelling feces (FSF) is human waste matter that has been stored in the colon and small intestine for a long time. It can cause CFS, fibromyalgia, confusion, depression, obesity, alcoholism, and death.

Foul-smelling feces is human waste matter that has been partly digested and left putrefying in the body. It creates *flatulence* and foul-smelling feces.

Rotting, putrefying waste matter in the colon and small intestine transmits toxins and breeds pathogens.

These things can cause CFS, fibromyalgia, chronic depression, confusion, brain fog, chronic illness, aches, pains, and even early death.

The idea that storing rotting, putrefying waste matter in the body is a leading cause of many illnesses is not readily understood by many medical doctors and other health practitioners.

Bernard Jensen, PhD, ND, did some amazing, groundbreaking work in this area.

His book, *Tissue Cleansing through Bowel Management*, should be read and studied by all persons who are seriously interested in healthy living and recovery.

53

FSF AND OBESITY: A CONNECTION

Rotting, putrefying waste matter that is being stored in the body is a prime breeding ground for toxic pathogens, such as excessive amounts of yeast and fungus. After these pathogens work themselves from the colon into the bloodstream, they can attack cells.

One defense used by cells against attack from pathogens is to become more rigid. They do this by retaining fluids. Just as a balloon that retains water, retaining liquid makes the outer membrane of the cell harder and thus less susceptible to invasion. However, *when the body retains fluids, it becomes heavier and obese.*

When the putrefying waste matter is removed from the colon and small intestine, yeast and fungus are reduced.

Then the cells retain less fluid.

As a result, the body loses weight and reduces in size.

54

FSF AND ALCOHOLISM

Rotting, putrefying waste matter stored in the body is a breeding ground for pathogens, such as excessive yeast and fungus.

As the yeast and fungus work themselves from the colon into the bloodstream, they attack the cells and organs and affect the brain. They attack and destroy sugar, which the brain needs to survive.

Some people who have an overload of fungus and yeast in their bodies have brains that demand that they use alcohol as its primary source of food as well as for their yeast and fungus. They are called *alcoholics*.

If those people removed the foul-smelling feces, which is the putrefying waste matter in their colons, they would also reduce the breeding ground for excessive yeast and fungus in their bodies, which causes them to crave alcohol.

For alcoholics, if they eliminated FSF, yeast and fungus would be reduced. The result would be that their cravings for alcohol would be reduced as well.

55

ANTIBIOTICS MAY HELP CHRONIC VIRAL INFECTIONS

Antibiotics kill bacteria. They do not kill viruses or infections caused by viruses, so doctors do not prescribe antibiotics for killing viral infections.

However, antibiotics may play a role in reducing viral infections. If there are many infections, including viral and bacterial infections, using antibiotics will reduce the amount of bacterial infections that the immune system must fight.

A reduction in the level of bacterial infections will increase the amount of energy available for the immune system to use to fight viral infections.

For those people who have an immune system that is not strong enough to kill enough viruses, it may be necessary to use antibiotics against their bacterial infections *in order to free up more energy* so that that energy can be used in the body's fight against their stubborn, overwhelming viral infections.

56

SOMETIMES ANTIBIOTICS MAY HELP RHEUMATOID ARTHRITIS

Many years ago, I met a nice older woman who was about eighty years old. She told me that she had suffered from severe rheumatoid arthritis in her hands for decades.

Her disease had become so bad, she said, that she could not use her hands to open doors by turning doorknobs. Instead, she said, she had to use her elbows.

She said her condition had become so intolerable that she had to seek help from a doctor in another country. He prescribed low doses of an antibiotic three days per week for three months.

As a result of that treatment, she showed me that she could use her hands to open doors by turning doorknobs.

I relay this story for those people who are victims of severe rheumatoid arthritis and who have found nothing else that works to remedy their illness.

57

Tests Dr. Shima and Others Performed On Me

1. Interro—a computer-generated testing program
2. Hair test for heavy metals
3. Hair test for mineral imbalances
4. Live blood-cell test
5. Mercury-vapor mouth test
6. Mercury-filling charge test
7. Heavy-metal absorption test using a chelating provocative agent
8. Pesticide absorption test
9. Poisoning from DDT and DDP
10. Poisoning from propyl alcohol
11. Poisoning from benzene
12. Poisoning from chlorine
13. Poisoning from fluoride
14. Essential fatty-acid absorption and imbalance tests
15. Omega-3 and omega-6 absorption tests

16. Free radical indication test

17. Mycoplasma tests

18. *Mycoplasma fermentans incognitus*

19. Giardia

20. Worms

21. Flukes and flatworms

22. Roundworms

23. Pinworms

24. Yeast

25. Candida

26. Fungus

27. STDs

28. HIV

29. Tuberculosis

30. Acidophilus

31. Vitamin D3 deficiency

32. Gut dysbiosis

33. Herpes

34. HHV-6

35. CMV

36. EBV

37. HPV

38. Lyme disease

39. Cancer

40. Celiac disease

41. Liver creatine clearing test

42. Lymph system tests

43. Colon tests
44. Digestion time clearance test
45. Hydrochloric acid test
46. Immune system test of NK cells
47. Immune system test, interleukin-6 and interleukin-10 tests
48. Tumor necrosis factor test
49. Brain damage using MRI and MRS tests
50. Thyroid tests—RTH, TSH
51. Pituitary tests—HGH
52. Testosterone test
53. Estrogen test
54. Adrenal test
55. Adrenal stress index test
56. Pancreatic enzyme
57. Urine pH
58. Saliva pH
59. Feces pH
60. Structural imbalance tests
61. Uneven weight distribution
62. Cranial misalignment
63. Spinal misalignment
64. Teeth balancing
65. Neurological testing
66. Leaky gut test
67. Hypoglycemia test
68. Fibromyalgia from Dr. R. Paul St. Amand

69. Asthma
70. Allergies
71. All vitamins
72. All minerals
73. All amino acids
74. Standard testing
75. Sjögren's syndrome

58

My Basic Road Map to Recovery

1. Remove heavy metals.
2. Remove toxic pesticides and herbicides.
3. Remove toxic waste matter.
4. Build up the immune system.
5. Reduce or eliminate pathogens such as yeast, fungus, mycoplasma, worms, flukes, bacteria, and viruses.
6. Repair and rebuild organs, tissues, and cells, such as liver, intestines, stomach, adrenals, kidneys, thyroid, pituitary, hypothalamus, pancreas, and lungs.
7. Repair the brain.
8. Repair the gut.
9. Reduce allergies.
10. Reduce asthma.
11. Reduce post-traumatic stress disorder.
12. Help others.
13. Surrender to Higher Power.

59

STAY EMPOWERED IN THE HEALING PROCESS

I have been very lucky. I had the money and the loving support from a devoted wife so I could go to many caring doctors, healers, dentists, naturopaths, and educated laypersons who guided me back from death's doorstep to life. Twenty-one years later, I am a much healthier, wiser, older man.

Twenty-one years ago, at the end of 1991, I was sleeping twenty hours a day and was in constant pain and in constant despair.

Now I sing, travel, write, ride a motorcycle, help others, and scuba dive. My transformation from being totally ill to returning to life has astounded my friends, my family, and myself.

The information in this book was gathered in so many ways from those who were so generous with their time, energy, knowledge, and wisdom during my recovery.

While I was traveling upon my "road to recovery," I learned some important lessons about the human body and the practice of medicine.

The following are some of the lessons I learned about being a patient in the United States:

Regarding remedies—everything works for somebody, but *not* everything works for everybody.

We are all different. We are all unique.

We all have a lot in common, but we all have a lot of differences.

My doctors and healers were my *consultants.*

They did not live in my body.

They saw me for only a brief period of time.

They had thousands of other patients to think about.

I learned that they could only make *quick* and *educated guesses* about my health issues.

I learned that I should *not expect* them to know a lot about me.

I learned that I *could not rely* exclusively on their judgments.

I learned that if I had doubts or I thought something was not going well, *it was up to me* to be more assertive.

I learned that *I had to make the final decision* about my health care because it was *my* body, *not* theirs.

I learned that *I had to take responsibility* for doing what I felt was right for me because it was my body, not theirs.

I learned that if something was not going right, then *I had to make a change.*

I learned that *I had to take charge of my health care.*

I learned that *I had to be proactive* in my health-care decisions.

I learned *I had to ask questions* such as

"What are the side effects?"

"When should I expect to see results?"

I learned that if a treatment wasn't working in a reasonable time, then it was time to *try something else.*

I learned that I had to *make my life an adventure, and regaining my health a challenge.*

I learned that the worst part of being sick in America is that our medical insurance system *does not provide enough money* for all the things I wanted to do.

I learned that *medical insurance is a very large problem* for most people with our illnesses.

Hopefully, this book will spur Congress and insurance companies to *provide additional funding* so doctors and healers can provide better testing and treatments for persons with these illnesses.

I learned that it *does not take much money* to get well once the *causes* of these illnesses are *found.*

60

EPILOGUE: SILVER LININGS

There were a few good things that came about because of Marc's illnesses and his "road to recovery."

First, because of the knowledge Marc gathered on his "road to recovery," he was able to give some people hope and a plan of action in their time of despair. For some, he was able to help them overcome their urge to commit suicide, get them to seek help from appropriate medical sources, and help them go on to live better, happier lives and enjoy major recoveries. He is very humbled and blessed for that honor.

Second, when Marc and his wife were visiting Israel in 1994, they saw that the Israelis were still using leaded gasoline. From his own personal struggle to overcome the toxic effects of lead poisoning, he understood quite clearly the kind of damage the Israelis were inflicting upon their children.

On his return to the United States, he wrote the Israeli leaders, reminding them of the dangers leaded gasoline posed to their children's health. Within a month, Israel began phasing out the use of leaded gasoline. Thank God for that one.

Third, during his recovery process, Marc came to understand that good food is required for recovery and healthy living. One day, he was visiting a dear friend who was recovering in a hospital in Ohio. He saw that the hospital was feeding his friend very unhealthy food.

On his return to San Diego, Marc wrote the hospital's directors and expressed his concerns. Once they realized that they could serve better quality food at no additional cost, they changed their ways. Again, Marc felt fortunate to have been a catalyst for constructive change.

If Marc had not become ill and had not been forced by his life's circumstances to spend so much time and effort learning about how to recover from his many illnesses, he is certain that he would not have been able to help (1) a few people overcome their despair and recover, (2) Israel begin using unleaded gasoline, and (3) a teaching hospital provide healthier food to its patients.

It is obvious that those blessings were directly related to and caused by Marc's recovery process.

Tikkun Olam.

61

About Marc S. Herlands, JD

Marc Herlands graduated from Shaker Heights High School near Cleveland, Ohio, in 1966; Tufts University near Boston, Massachusetts, in 1970; Georgetown University Law Center in Washington, DC, in 1973; and he earned a master's degree in tax law from the University of San Diego, California, in 1987.

In April 1974, Marc began the practice of law in an eastern suburb of Cleveland, Ohio. In November 1974, at the age of twenty-six, he had his first major attack of chronic fatigue syndrome. By February 1975, he had to stop practicing law full-time because he was so tired, slept poorly, was constantly exhausted, was emotionally upset, depressed, and constantly hungry. His doctor told him he was "burned out," and he had to rest.

From 1975 through 1991 (ages twenty-seven to forty-three), Marc passed all his standard medical tests, but no one could tell him why he was sleeping over twenty hours per day or why he couldn't sleep without narcotics—since his fibromyalgia pain was so horrible it kept him awake at night.

Beginning in late 1991, his doctor, dentist, and other healers began to discover the causes of his health problems. They slowly discovered the causes of his chronic fatigue syndrome, fibromyalgia, Gulf War syndrome, heavy-metal toxicity, depression, chronic yeast infection, mycoplasma infection, obesity, internal alcoholism, celiac disease, immune system dysfunction, enzyme deficiency, leaky gut syndrome, and other maladies—all of which are revealed in this book.

This is the story of how Marc discovered with his doctors, healers, and wife the mysterious, underlying causes of his illnesses, and how he miraculously recovered his health over many decades using many unconventional methods to become an author, attorney, loving husband, caregiver, singer, world traveler, and scuba diver.

During his recovery, he was co-chair of the Chronic Fatigue Syndrome and Fibromyalgia Research and Support Group of San Diego, California, with Ms. Jo Nost for more than five years in the 1990s. The group had more than four hundred members, most of whom had CFS and fibromyalgia, but a few were their supporters and caregivers.

Marc's recovery is remarkable because his brain and most of his bodily systems were substantially impaired.

Along his "road to recovery," Marc made some amazing personal and medical discoveries while answering some very basic questions, which had gone unanswered by his primary doctors for over seventeen years:

1. Why am I ill?
2. What can I do about it?

He wrote this book because he wants to help the people who suffer from the same illnesses he did.

He wants them to receive the kind of care—or better—from their doctors, dentists, healers, medical consultants, caregivers, family, friends, and support system that he did on his road to recovery.

Simply put, he wants them to have the information that helped him recover from his illnesses—but faster and with less pain and suffering.

62

About Dr. Gary J. Shima, MD

Dr. Gary J. Shima graduated from Arcadia High School in Arcadia, California, in 1958; University of Southern California in Los Angeles, California, as an undergraduate in 1961, and from their medical school in 1965. He was board certified in family medicine and has been a practicing medical doctor in California since 1968.

Beginning in 1981, Dr. Shima began an active medical practice that emphasized preventive health care for patients located in various board and care facilities throughout San Diego County. In 1987, he became a California State medical consultant for medical care at board and care facilities throughout the State of California.

In 1990, Dr. Shima became the director and service physician at the Comprehensive Medical Center (now known as Center for Advanced Medicine) in Encinitas, California, where he specialized in treating patients with chronic illnesses, the causes of which were not apparent, and the treatments were not obvious.

At CMC, Dr. Shima began to include alternative and complementary medicine treatments to augment his standard medical protocols. He started using nutritionists, chiropractors, and others to help his chronically ill patients heal better and faster when more traditional treatments and remedies did not produce satisfactory results in a cost-effective or timely manner.

In 1996, Dr. Shima became the director and service physician at the Health and Longevity Institute in Vista, California. That institute is now located in San Marcos, California. He now specializes in anti-aging medicine and hormone replacement therapy.

At the age of seventy-three, he is physically and mentally fit, very active and strong, maintains a medical practice, plays baseball, travels, and is close to his family and grandchildren.

For More Information

For additional books, e-books, and other products as they become available, please visit our website at

www.artofhealingbook.com

Contact the authors at

artofhealingbook@gmail.com

Thank you very much

for reading our book.

We wish you
good luck, good health, and
Godspeed.

Dr. Gary J. Shima

Marc S. Herlands

Index

V

vanadium, 19, 32, 66, 96, 98, 101
viral infections, 18, 65, 166, 194-95
vitamins, 9, 15, 18, 33-34, 56, 126,
    154, 159, 201

W

waste matter, 113, 117-18
Watson, Roxanne, 27, 30, 108
weapon of mass destruction, 33,
    67, 174
weight, 59-60, 155, 178-79, 191
whiplash, 127, 156-57
worms, 67, 199, 202

Y

yeast, 9, 20, 33, 56-58, 60, 67, 94,
    119, 126, 138, 142-44, 173,
    180-87, 190-93, 199

List of References

Chronic Fatigue Syndrome and Fibromyalgia

Detoxify or Die by Sherry A. Rogers, M.D.

From Fatigued to Fantastic by Jacob Teitelbaum, M.D.

Tired or Toxic? A Blueprint for Health by Sherry A. Rogers, M.D.

Yeast and Fungus

The Fungus Link to Health Problems by Douglas A. Kaufmann

The Yeast Connection and Women's Health by William G. Crook, M.D.

Heavy Metal Toxicity

The Complete Guide to Mercury Toxicity from Dental Fillings by Joyal Taylor, D.D.S.

It's All in Your Head: The Link Between Mercury Amalgams and Illness by Hal A. Huggins, M.D.

Toxic Metal Syndrome by H. Richard Casdorph, M.D. and Morton Walker, M.D.

Depression

Ageless: Take Control of Your Age and Stay Youthful for Life by Edward L. Schneider, M.D. and Elizabeth Miles

The Instinct to Heal: Curing Depression, Anxiety, and Stress Without Drugs and Without Talk Therapy by David Servan-Schreiber, M.D., PhD

Nutrition

The Healing Foods: The Ultimate Authority on the Curative Power of Nutrition by Patricia Hausman and Judith Benn Hurley

The Missing Link: In the Medical Curriculum: Which Is Food Chemistry . . . by Jay M. Hoffman, M.D.